# How to Complete a PhD in the Medical and Clinical Sciences

T0201162

# How to Complete a PhD in the Medical and Clinical Sciences

**Edited by**

**Ashton Barnett-Vanes**
St George's, University of London and Imperial College London, UK

**Rachel Allen**
Reader in Immunology of Infection and Head of Graduate School
St George's, University of London, UK

WILEY Blackwell

# Contents

# List of contributors

**Kyrillos N Adesina-Georgiadis DIC PhD**
Honorary Research Associate
Imperial College London
UK

**Rachel Allen DPhil**
Reader in Immunology of Infection and Head of Graduate School
St George's, University of London
UK

**Ashton Barnett-Vanes BSc PhD**
MB-PhD Candidate
St George's, University of London and Imperial College London
UK

**Adel Benlahrech PhD**
Post-doctoral researcher
University of Oxford
UK

**Manu Chhabra MBBChir PhD**
Doctor
National University Hospital, Singapore and University of Cambridge
Singapore, UK

**Timothy M Cox FMedSci**
Emeritus Professor of Medicine and Director of Research
University of Cambridge
UK

**Fiona Cunningham BSc PhD**
Professor of Pharmacology
Royal Veterinary College
UK

**Henry D.I. De'Ath PhD MRCS**
Surgical Registrar and Honorary Clinical Lecturer
Wessex Deanery and Queen Mary, University of London
UK

**Michael Dustin PhD**
Professor of Immunology
University of Oxford
UK

**Jonathan Elliott PhD MRCVS**
Professor of Veterinary Clinical Pharmacology and
Vice Principal for Research and Innovation
Royal Veterinary College
UK

**Kate Gowers PhD**
Research Associate
University College London
UK

**E. Allison Green BSc PhD FHEA**
Senior Lecturer
University of York
UK

**Ming He MBBS MRCS PhD**
Surgical Research Fellow
Imperial College London and King's College Hospital
UK

**Rebecca Ingram PhD PGCHET**
Lecturer
Queen's University Belfast
UK

**Laura Lambert MA PhD**
Post-doctoral researcher
Imperial College London
UK

**Paul Langford BSc PhD**
Professor of Paediatric Infectious Diseases
Imperial College London
UK

**Jonathan C.H. Lau BSc MSc**
MB-PhD Candidate
University of Cambridge and University College London
UK

**Fiona Reid BSc MSc**
Senior Lecturer in Statistics
King's College London and St George's, University of London
UK

**David Salman MBBS MCRP**
Wellcome Trust Clinical Research Training Fellow
Imperial College London
UK

**Célia A. Soares MD**
MD-PhD Candidate
School of Health Sciences, University of Minho
Portugal

**John Tregoning MA PhD**
Senior Lecturer
Imperial College London
UK

**Fiona Tomley BSc PhD**
Professor of Experimental Parasitology
Royal Veterinary College
UK

**Kristien Verheyen PhD MRCVS**
Senior Lecturer in Clinical Epidemiology and Head of Graduate School
Royal Veterinary College
UK

**Andrew John Walley MA DPhil**
Senior Lecturer in Human Genomics
St George's, University of London
UK

# About the editors

Dr Ashton Barnett-Vanes is an MB-PhD Candidate based in London. He completed his medical and clinical science years at St George's, University of London where he was awarded the William Brown and Devitt-Pendlebury Exhibition. In 2012, he graduated with First Class Honours in his intercalated BSc and in 2015 completed his PhD in War Injuries, both at Imperial College London. In 2016, he was a British Council Scholar at Tsinghua University, Beijing. He is the recipient of a Foulkes Foundation Fellowship. Read more at www.howtophd.com   @HowtoPhD

Dr Rachel Allen is a Reader in Immunology of Infection at St George's, University of London. She obtained her DPhil in Immunology at the Weatherall Institute of Molecular Medicine in Oxford and was awarded a Beit Memorial Fellowship to continue her postdoctoral studies at Cambridge University. In addition to her research activities (including PhD supervision) since joining St George's in 2007, Rachel has acted as Associate Dean for Research Degrees and was appointed Head of the Graduate School in 2014.

# Foreword

Episodic evolution of health care within the modern state and explosive progress in science have had transformative effects on medicine; but human nature has changed little and people still fall ill! While many formerly intractable diseases can now be treated or prevented, it is a striking fact that nearly all therapeutic advances have been developed and introduced by scientifically minded researchers and doctors. The distinctive mind-set of those who materially advance understanding or introduce successful cures, is usually characterised as that most favourable for scientific thinking: insatiable curiosity; strong ideals; an often irritating and a sceptical mistrust of hand-me-down explanations of natural phenomena – and distaste for rote learning.

Today's research climate presents myriad challenges and opportunities for the next cadre of researchers. Doctors Ashton Barnett-Vanes and Rachel Allen bring a complementary perspective to this field: intimately familiar with the demands, conflicts and practicalities of the clinical research universe, their scientific perspectives are broad and their experiences deep; their advice is realistic. Here they have collected a set of frank chapters from like-minded authors that offer an excellent conspectus of the opportunities, pitfalls and sheer diversity of activities that make up the fascinating science that clinical undergraduates, graduates in medicine and allied clinical sciences are eligible to pursue.

The path of the clinical investigator has been well trodden throughout history. Nonetheless, all that we know and apply now for the relief of human suffering has depended on understanding gained by a relatively few great experimenters from the past. To meet its societal obligations, contemporary medicine remains dependent on the engagement of imaginative scientists and clinicians who can make and introduce discoveries into clinical practice and public health. Proportionately, these people are likely to be ever fewer representatives of our profession: for those launching themselves onto this path with research formalised into PhD programmes, I commend this intriguing and helpful collection. Direct, informative, practical: it is, above all, encouraging!

Timothy M Cox, FMedSci
*Emeritus Professor of Medicine and Director of Research*
*Founding Director, MB-PhD programme*
*University of Cambridge, UK*

# Preface

Deciding and embarking upon a 3–4-year period of exploration is easy to be excited about. But with exploration comes uncertainty: will I get enough data? What will my lab group be like? Will I make a scientific break-through and/or find a cure? Could I inundate PubMed?

As a PhD student in a world class research institute, I both witnessed and experienced the great spectrum of outcomes that greet those undertaking a PhD. From the student with enough data to write their thesis in the first year, to the student starting their final year without any convincing results.

This book is written for current and prospective PhD students in the medical and clinical sciences. It seeks, through concise chapters, to help provide a framework and guidance for students of all training backgrounds (scientific or clinical) to complete their PhD and move on. It cannot be understated how far-fetched the phrase 'complete and move on' can seem to most PhD students at one time or another. But, out of darkness cometh light. We hope this book will help illuminate that path.

Dr Ashton Barnett-Vanes

Committing several years of your life to a single piece of work is a major decision. Nobody will ever undertake the same PhD project in the same way as you, so it will be a step into the unknown. This book is intended to help you steer yourself to one known outcome – the award of a Doctoral degree.

As a PhD student, then supervisor, then Head of Graduate School I've seen that, despite the unique nature of each PhD, there are many common experiences for PhD students. This book combines the advice of PhD students and academics on how to navigate the various stages of the degree; how to prepare, what to expect and what to do when some- (or every-) thing seems to be going wrong. We hope that this will prepare you for every stage of your PhD, saving the surprises for your research.

Dr Rachel Allen

# Acknowledgements

I thank my co-editor Rachel Allen for her unwavering support for this book and its aims; Dr George Hall and Dr Suman Rice for helpful discussions and advice during the genesis of this project; James Watson, our commissioning editor at Wiley, for his support from the beginning of this book and Loan Nguyen, Yogalakshmi Mohanakrishnan, Lynette Woodward, Rajitha Selvarajan and Thaatcher Missier Glen at Wiley for their advice and assistance throughout the production and editing process. My thanks to students and colleagues who wittingly or otherwise gave me inspiration for this project. Finally, I owe a debt of gratitude to friends and family whose patience and generosity enabled me to take this book to completion.

Dr Ashton Barnett-Vanes

I'd like to thank all the authors who contributed to this book, for their enthusiasm and insights into the PhD experience – it's been a great opportunity for us to learn from each other. In particular, I'd like to express thanks to my co-editor Ashton, who conceived the original idea for this book and acted as motivator-in-chief to keep the project on course.

Dr Rachel Allen

# Chapter 1 **Introduction**

*Ashton Barnett-Vanes[1] and Rachel Allen[2]*

[1] MB-PhD Candidate, St George's, University of London and Imperial College London, UK

[2] Reader in Immunology of Infection and Head of Graduate School, St George's, University of London, UK

## A PhD

Well done on picking up (and ideally purchasing!) this book. If you're considering or about to embark on a PhD in the clinical and medical sciences, or related life/natural science disciplines, this might be one of the last scientific books you purchase. That's not because it's so good as to *end* all others, or that it's so outrageously bad you go off books altogether; but because PhDs are about new knowledge, books are about old knowledge – with new diagrams. That said, why is this book worth reading? Well, before we get to that, it's worth first laying out the PhD landscape that awaits you.

A large amount of UK research is publicly funded. You know the drill – law abiding citizens work and pay taxes, which are then distributed around our economy. Now, as well as subsidising first class seats on empty trains, some of this money goes into big productive industries, including science. Medical research charities are another major source of science funding, along with the pharmaceutical industry and related enterprises. In the UK, about 1.5% of GDP is invested in research and development[(1)]; the two largest of these funders of scientific/medical research – the Medical Research Council and the Wellcome Trust – collectively spend just over £1 billion per year. That's a lot of money, enough to buy 167 000 hip replacements, 22 000 teachers or four (Challenger) battle tanks[(2)]. This money filters down a scientific waterfall and finds its way into universities, research institutes, laboratory groups, and occasionally PhD student bar tabs – sorry, projects. At any one time, there are around 30 000 PhD students in: medicine and dentistry, subjects allied to medicine, biological sciences and veterinary science[(3)]; which to give you a sense of scale is about the same population as Gibraltar...

*How to Complete a PhD in the Medical and Clinical Sciences,*
First Edition. Edited by Ashton Barnett-Vanes and Rachel Allen.
© 2018 John Wiley & Sons Ltd. Published 2018 by John Wiley & Sons Ltd.

To wrap this up, it's worth knowing that each PhD student is quite an investment. A three-year stipend will reach around £45 000; a consumables budget could easily reach £30 000, not to mention those tuition fees. In short, each PhD student costs around £100 000, that's £2.7 Billion of coinage going into one cohort of PhD students, lots of which comes from the public and charitable sectors; moreover, this cost can be significantly higher when considering clinical trainees undertaking a PhD. There's also the time invested in the enterprise by your supervisors, and their equivalent salary costs. While 3 or 4 years sounds like a long time (and it kind of is!), this is comparatively short compared to other countries. For example, PhDs in the United States can sometimes double that duration. So, if we're going to keep 'our' PhDs comparatively shorter, safeguard their international prestige, ensure they're value for money – and actually have a good chance of discovering something; it's vital that projects are conducted efficiently and effectively from the get go. That's where this book comes in.

## Perspective

Research is exciting. The focus and expertise you can acquire on a specific area is quite incredible, at times even alarming. On this relatively solitary journey, it's easy to feel you're in the know, and everyone else isn't, but keep perspective. Check the illustrations below for what we're getting at, courtesy of Matt Might[4].

Imagine this circle represents the boundaries of human knowledge, everything we know is contained within it.

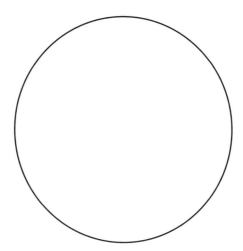

**Figure 1.1** Courtesy of Dr Matt Might

The circles represent different levels of human knowledge, the inner circle is what we learn in primary school, they expand into secondary school and begin to reach out as Bachelors, Masters and eventually PhDs – the latter furrowing at the edges of human understanding.

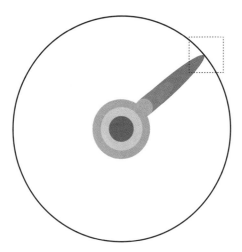

**Figure 1.2**

Here's what your PhD looks like to you, as you push against the wall of current knowledge.

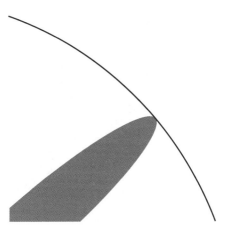

**Figure 1.3**

Eventually you'll make your mark, and push that boundary forwards – expanding human knowledge.

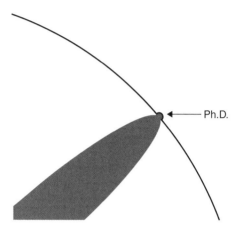

**Figure 1.4**

Here's how it looks to you up close as the researcher.

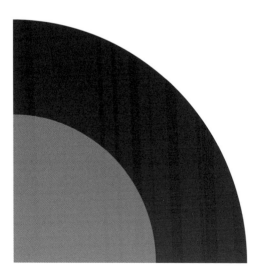

**Figure 1.5**

But remember, this is how it looks to everyone else.

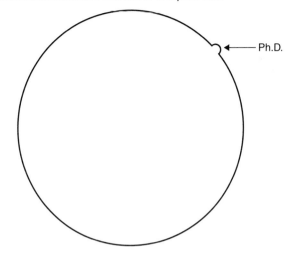

Ph.D.

**Figure 1.6**

## Why a book? How to use it

There are ample books to help students get through their undergraduate studies; get a 'First' or write a good Master's thesis and so on. But oddly, when it comes to the highest degree on offer in the UK, books offering guidance on PhDs are all too often generic, with some even as long as a doctoral thesis! Of course, you should receive a student handbook from your university, but these are seldom an inspiring read or source of friendly advice. This book addresses these shortcomings three-fold. First, it's aimed at a much narrower audience, focusing on medical and clinical science PhDs, and related bio-medical and life-science disciplines. Second, it is direct and concise; PhD students can often be overwhelmed by the amount of literature reading they need to do, a guide book should be there to support not supplant. Third, this book combines the perspectives of current or recent PhD graduates with those of senior researchers, from both scientific and clinical backgrounds. We hope that this will give you an insight into academic's expectations, while avoiding the potential for a 'how it was in my day' bias.

While you're welcome to use this book anyway you want, we recommend its use 'on the go'. Some chapters will be suitable for specific time points such as the Year 1–3 chapters; others for specific situations, such as when finding a PhD or writing a paper; and some chapters will have a continuous relevance, such as dealing with problems or delivering a presentation. If you're not a medical or clinical science PhD student, don't put us down just yet. Though that's our primary audience, this book will work for anyone doing a PhD in scientific research in a laboratory or clinical department. While we focus on PhDs throughout, this book will equally be suitable to those clinical researchers undertaking 'MDRes' degrees; the only main difference is the potentially shortened time frame for active research, which arguably makes this book even more indispensable.

Finally, alongside the bread and butter chapters you'd expect, we've included a couple extras. The international PhD chapter reflects the increasing international connectivity among research projects, opening up new opportunities for PhD students. The Post-doc and Professor chapters offer insight into career routes and senior researcher perspectives – we ask the awkward questions so you don't have to.

So, without further ado, welcome, happy reading and good luck!

## References

1. EUROSTAT Europe 2020 indicators - research and development, available online at http://ec.europa.eu/eurostat/statistics-explained/index.php/Europe_2020_indicators_-_research_and_development (accessed 8 December, 2016).
2. BBC News Magazine article, Election 2015: What does a billion pounds actually buy the nation? Tom Castella. Available online at: www.bbc.co.uk/news/magazine-32309311 (accessed 8 December, 2016).
3. Higher Education Statistics Agency, data and analysis, available online at: https://www.hesa.ac.uk/stats (accessed 8 December, 2016).
4. Might, M. *The Illustrated Guide to a PhD*. Available online at http://matt.might.net/articles/phd-school-in-pictures/(accessed 8 December, 2016).

# Chapter 2  **Deciding on and finding a PhD**

*Jonathan C.H. Lau[1] and Ming He[2]*

[1] MB-PhD Candidate, University of Cambridge and University College London, UK

[2] Surgical Research Fellow, Imperial College London and King's College Hospital, UK

## Background

Applying for a PhD project is one of the first and most crucial steps of your academic journey. It sets you on a PhD path that, if chosen wisely, should be not only be secure, feasible and motivating; but above all, worthwhile and productive. A good project, one that fosters such attributes, will help to offset the difficulties and challenges that you may come to face, while also granting maximal opportunity to reap several important benefits – be it getting a first author publication, travelling abroad to attend conferences, striking lifelong friendships and future collaborations, or indeed, simply succeeding in taking the work from conception through to completion (a noble endeavour in itself).

Quite unsurprisingly, therefore, the task of choosing a project to embark on, with all that it entails – the supervisor(s), research theme, affiliated university/institution, mode of funding, timeliness and so on – may seem daunting. Moreover, there is also likely to be fierce competition for any doctoral position. Nevertheless, efforts to overcome these hurdles should be channelled accordingly to help reach a firm decision, one that reflects your own preferences for what an 'ideal' project should be or consist of. While there is no such thing as a perfect project, it is well within your means to find a project that ultimately suits you; however, this requires your proactive participation.

Medical and clinical science projects vary in their nature, with some already having funded proposals in place. Such projects, which are 'ready to go', tend to have a more structured feel to the application process. However, these projects are often less flexible in what they may offer you in scope, compared to a project that you co-develop with a prospective supervisor.

*How to Complete a PhD in the Medical and Clinical Sciences,*
First Edition. Edited by Ashton Barnett-Vanes and Rachel Allen.
© 2018 John Wiley & Sons Ltd. Published 2018 by John Wiley & Sons Ltd.

Consequently, it is common for medical science PhD applicants to prepare multiple applications for a range of suitable projects, or alternatively, for institutions to offer a choice on potential projects once a place has been awarded. This contrasts with higher degrees in the arts and humanities, where project proposals may frequently be written and thus tailored from scratch.

The aim of this chapter is to detail the process of applying for a PhD and provide a sensible strategy for selecting a project and securing it.

## Routes of entry

Deciding when in your career to apply for a PhD is largely dictated by your career track: scientific or clinical.

The scientific route typically progresses from an undergraduate Bachelor's degree (e.g. BSc), on to a Master's degree or directly to a PhD. A Bachelor's degree in any aspect of medical or clinical science is likely to contain a research project; serving as the first opportunity to develop an understanding of research methods and build a relationship with researchers in a specific field. It's important you achieve strongly in this Bachelor's, with ideally at least a 2:1 honours degree. Master's projects may take the form of taught courses with a research component (MSc) or a research-focused degree often with several research rotations (MRes). Alternatively, an MSc degree will provide you with a ~4-year rounded education in science, gaining a Masters qualification on an undergraduate funding system. Either way, achieving a merit or distinction in your Master's degree is necessary if you are to make a strong PhD application.

Again, alongside developing scientific research skills, these degrees and research programmes provide a platform to engage with researchers and senior academics to raise your profile above the competition as a prospective PhD candidate. Presenting or publishing during your time as a Bachelor's or Master's student (see Chapter 8) is likely to strengthen your perceived suitability for a position; it will also garner support (such as references or letters of support) from colleagues, improving your competitiveness in applying elsewhere. Finally, if you're lacking a Master's, an alternative way to boost your CV is to demonstrate a track record of research experience, for example as a research assistant in a laboratory (see Chapter 3) – but along this route, you risk being 'outgunned' by those with stronger academic qualifications, irrespective of research assistant time.

### Clinical track
Over the last decade, the implementation of the National Institute of Health Research integrated academic training programme has enabled would be academic trainees to incorporate both clinical and academic

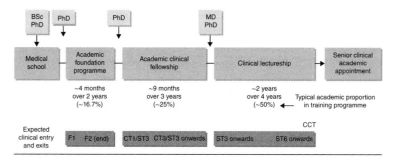

**Figure 2.1** Career routes in academic medicine. Courtesy of Dr Garth Funston/*BMJ Careers*

training simultaneously (see Figure 2.1). Beginning at medical school and continuing after qualification, this flexible framework has become the mainstay for clinical academic training in the UK, providing multiple possible entry points for acquiring a PhD, while also enabling resumption of clinical training or ongoing career progression. Although all routes of entry culminate in the award of a doctorate, not all necessarily share the same structure or composition in terms of duration, entry requirements, pay bands, ongoing professional development, and protected time allocation for research. Consequently, with each one having its own merits and drawbacks, certain routes may appeal more to some than to others and thus require careful consideration.

Along the clinical academic career path, one may embark on their PhD at two broadly different possible time points or routes:
1. Pre-qualification PhD ('MB-PhD') route
2. Post-qualification PhD route

**Pre-qualification route**
Of all possible entry points for those on a clinical track, the pre-qualification PhD ('MB-PhD') route represents the earliest opportunity to obtain a PhD while also attaining a primary medical qualification (MBBS or equivalent). It is the UK equivalent of the 'MD-PhD' programme, which was first established in the USA more than 40 years ago. Presently, few UK medical schools offer formal MB/PhD programmes including the University of Cambridge and University College London.

The key requirement to undertake an MB-PhD is having (or committing to attain) an intercalated BSc (iBSc), often with upper second class or first honours. Applications for MB-PhD programmes typically occur in the year prior to starting clinical training; for 5-year MBBS courses, this corresponds to the year leading up to the award of an iBSc; while for 4-year graduate entry programmes, this corresponds to the second year of pre-clinical training. In general, most students on their MB-PhD programme start by following their school's clinical curriculum for the first 24 or so months, before diverting into a period of full-time research that paves the way to the PhD itself. Alongside formal programmes, it is also possible as a medical student to self-organise a PhD, through an 'interruption of studies' organised with your university, and apply directly for PhD studentships alongside other science track students.

The difference between formal and self-intercalated projects can be significant. Formal programmes are likely to have a more fixed timeline with introductions and PhD projects offered directly to students, with typically a few hours each week devoted to ongoing clinical education and bedside teaching. Self-intercalated PhDs may not have these benefits, however, the greater autonomy over your project and schedule may still appeal. Once students have successfully completed their PhD, they return to where they left off by re-joining their clinical course at the start of the appropriate year. Doing a PhD during medical school is slightly more flexible than embarking on one after (see later). Here, you won't have clinical rotas/responsibilities you're contractually obliged to return to – should your PhD run into difficulties that may necessitate an additional 6–12 months of research time.

## Post-qualification PhD route

Qualified medics who are fully registered with the GMC have the option of integrating a PhD into the middle of their training, usually with the intention of embarking on a career as a clinical academic. Those wishing to do so are strongly encouraged to follow the academic career path and apply for positions within the academic foundation programme (AFP) and/or academic clinical fellowship (ACF), which feature as distinct run-through training posts for the Foundation Programme and early stages of speciality training (i.e. ST1 core medical training), respectively. These schemes provide ringfenced research time, conferring additional academic training opportunities that can aid in preparing and applying for a PhD, while also enabling trainees to continue practising and maintaining their clinical skills. While the importance of clinical academic training posts in helping to secure a place on a PhD programme – which includes funding – are significant; having one is not a prerequisite to making a PhD application. Indeed, several doctors have successfully applied for PhDs without having either had a place on the AFP or a ACF – though, in such cases, individuals would still have likely acquired research experience before preparing their application.

Once a PhD has begun, doctors will devote their time accordingly over the next 3 or 4 years (if full-time and longer if part-time) to complete their work. During this period, however, they will have the opportunity to maintain and develop their clinical skills by participating in on call rotas, clinics and/or medical teaching. Most PhDs begun by this particular route usually occur after around 5 years post-qualification training, but may happen earlier (e.g. following foundation training). Once this has been completed and the final degree awarded, doctors will resume their normal clinical duties, moving forwards with their speciality training/career progression. Note, that this transition is usually fixed and inflexible – occasionally doctors undertaking PhDs find themselves rushing or not completing their final research experiments due to the resumption of full clinical responsibilities. Planning way in advance and being realistic with your research objectives are therefore crucial.

In summary, the options for those on a scientific track wishing to pursue a PhD are clear; to embark on one immediately after a Bachelor's degree (rare) or after further completion of a Master's degree. For those on a clinical track, the picture is more complex. In undertaking a PhD early (MB-PhD), students develop research skills that can be applied throughout their clinical training. However, they risk undertaking a project that may not match their ultimate clinical ambitions. Undertaking a PhD later in clinical training may offer students the chance to better match their research with clinical interests, however, the demands and competing clinical commitments on students such as on-calls and teaching, can reduce the time available for uninterrupted research; though qualified doctors undergoing PhDs receive a valuable clinical salary to reflect this added burden compared to the more modest research stipend available to MB-PhD students (discussed next).

While each entry route may ultimately influence the choice of projects available, each potential project should still be judged accordingly by its own merits; and this consideration alone should ideally be the key factor in deciding whether to pursue a particular project – as the following section 2.3 will now describe.

## How to find one

Whether on a scientific or clinical track, in considering how to apply for a PhD you should already have some idea of which institution(s) you wish to consider. Here, we'll focus on those wishing to apply within the UK, for those considering an international PhD see Chapter 11.

PhDs may be offered directly by university departments; major research funders (such as the Wellcome Trust of Medical Research Council); by major institutes such as the Francis Crick, or together in partnership. Identifying opportunities early is vital. This can be through official channels of advertising such as university webpages and search pages like www.findaphd.com, or

**Box 2.1** Popular websites/for a listing PhD projects

- University websites
- Research lab websites
- www.postgraduatestudentships.co.uk
- www.Findaphd.com
- Learned societies

through more personal 'networked' channels such as LinkedIn; the growing network of Doctoral Training Partnerships and centres are another avenue to examine (see Box 2.1). Finally, keep an eye out on the webpages of suitable research labs and their principle investigators as they occasionally advertise opportunities directly through these mediums – ensuring only students with a keen interest in their work apply.

A place to start is by considering what field you wish to undertake a PhD in. Different universities and research institutes have particular research strengths. For example, if you're passionate about trauma research, London (with five major trauma centres and several research centres) might be the place for you. Besides the institutional strengths, factor in your existing location or areas of interest. City-based projects will have different experiences academically and socially to town-based projects. If you're in a city, are you centrally based (e.g. King's College London) or a suburb (e.g. University of Roehampton). Consider factors like cost of living and travel; are you willing to commute long-distance? Lab based or clinical projects can often have unsocial hours: is there a night bus or will your laboratory pay taxi expenses when there's no public transport?

PhD programmes are often specific to the institution or department's interests and skill sets, in order to provide specialist supervision. Supervisors will have a range of potential projects and it's advisable to approach them early to discuss what might be on offer or in the pipeline. While most are approachable (few supervisors are offended by an enthusiastic, well-phrased and concise email), it's prudent to contact current students in the department to gauge their experience and perspectives.

Tours of the department or laboratory are a common vehicle to achieve this. As an unwritten rule, if a student does not enthusiastically recommend you join – take note; students will never want to bad mouth their supervisor or department to outsiders, but subtle signs might be on show. If you're concerned, simple questions like asking what the turnover of staff is or how often they see their supervisor might provide some insight.

## Choosing a project

You have now arrived at an exciting venture: the time to choose a project for your PhD. By this stage, you should already have an idea about the field of research you would like to go into and the potential locations. Deciding upon a project that best suits your interests is not an easy task. Most on offer will appear likeable, and with each one being presented in a positive light – vying for the attention of potential applicants – it can be difficult to distinguish strong projects from weak ones. Moreover, it's important to consider what kind of supervisor you'd work best with for (at least) 3 years. Thus, in choosing a project it's vital to probe carefully before reaching a final decision to avoid disappointment (or in some cases shock) further down the line.

Discussing projects face to face with potential supervisors is the most effective way of learning about them. However, as it is impractical to arrange a meeting with every potential group, it is important to start by creating a shortlist of projects that may be suitable. Afterwards, supervisors from each shortlisted project may be contacted in turn to arrange a visit in-person. To help with this overall process of creating a shortlist, and finalising your decision, two separate checklists have been devised respectively for you to follow – each one containing a useful set of questions to help guide your decision as well as advise you on where to look for more information.

### Checklist I: Shortlisting potential PhD projects

A.  Is your desired theme or topic of research on offer?
   - Consult different university departments across the UK, particularly if they are already advertising funded PhD programmes in key areas of research, such as cancer (e.g. Cancer Research UK) or infection (e.g. Wellcome Trust)
   - Visit individual research group webpages from various universities or affiliated research institutions (e.g. NIMR) and enquire if they are willing to consider individual applications from prospective PhD students
   - If project descriptions are not available, see if the group describes what lines of investigation they are actively pursuing
B.  Will the project employ methodologies that you are interested in using yourself?
   - See what research techniques are typically performed by the group (i.e. is it laboratory based, computer-based, clinically orientated, or multi-disciplinary)
   - If the group specialises solely in a particular research technique, check whether they regularly collaborate with other groups that employ different research techniques

C.  What is the research output of each group like?
  • Look at the groups' webpages and go through publications (both recent and historical) – if publications are not listed, then perform a PubMed search of the supervisor
  • See if there is a steady turnover of publications in well-known, established journals (*EMBO*, *PNAS*, *PLoS*, *J Exp Med*, *J Virol* etc.) and/or high impact journals (*Nature*, *Science*, *Cell*, *NEJM* etc.)
D.  What are the perceived dynamics of the group?
  • Look at the size and composition of the group – is it small (<10 members) or large (>10 members), and how many PhD students, academic staff (e.g. research associates and/or readers) and support staff (e.g. research assistants) does it have?
  • Check if the work is headed either by an established senior member of staff or perhaps a young, but 'up-and-coming' individual
E.  Aside from the research group, what are other factors like, for instance the choice of university?
  • With regards to choosing a project in general, most weighting should be given to the group itself rather than to any other factor; however, for some applicants, the choice of university may also be important for other reasons
  • Check that your chosen university provide sufficient opportunities to engage in clinical work, especially if you intend to integrate your PhD with ongoing clinical practice
  • Collegiate universities, such as Oxford, Cambridge and Durham, operate on a very different system to most others in the UK, in which most activities – be it sporting or social and so on – are organised by separate colleges rather than centrally through the university itself.

## Checklist II: Finalising your decision on a PhD project
A.  Can you get along with your supervisor as well as the group as a whole?
  • Speak openly with the supervisor about your aspirations in working with the group, making sure that he/she is sympathetic to your goals
  • Enquire if your supervisor will be readily available to discuss work or other matters in-person, or alternatively will delegate this particular role to another member staff who you are able to get along well with
  • Wherever possible, speak to current members of the group (especially current PhD students) and ask for their own opinion about working there; cross-check their responses with those of the prospective supervisor
  • Ascertain if the group follows a particular work ethic, which may feature a mixture of styles (e.g. hard-working or relaxed, independent or closely supervised etc.), and consider if this is compatible for you in the long run

B. Will this project be productive and worthwhile?
  - As a primary goal, check with the supervisor if he/she aims to ensure that your PhD will result in the publication of at least one first author paper in a respectable journal (this is usually expected from most PhD students)
  - Look at the groups' listed publications and check how many first- and/ or co-authors are PhD students
  - Ask if the supervisor organises regular trips to conferences (including ones that are abroad) and actively encourages PhD students to submit abstracts for oral presentations as well as poster presentations
C. Is this project at risk of major or sudden setbacks?
  - Double-check your own position in relation to the project prior to applying, in particular, whether you will need to secure any funding yourself (in which case, it is worth asking if the group will be able to help you) or if funding is already in place (e.g. the group is in possession of a studentship)
  - Additionally, check that the group itself is already in possession of its own funding or has recently had its own grant(s) renewed and is therefore financially secure and is not leaving pressure on its students to provide money
  - Make sure that your supervisor or anyone likely to be involved with your day-to-day supervision is not scheduled to leave or sever ties with the group until you are settled in – in some cases, this cannot be avoided (e.g. some may go on parental leave), but direct contact can still be established and is not on par with exiting staff taking up a new job/ position elsewhere
D. Will potential conflict arise between you and any other current PhD students or staff members?
  - In most cases, it will not be possible to meet everyone in the group (let alone those who may join in the future), but it is important to meet enough to help leave you with an impression of what working there is like
  - If multiple PhD students will be joining the group at the same time, check that each student will be tasked to different areas of research that are distinct from each other, having little or no overlap
E. Outside the laboratory, what are the opportunities for socialising and doing extracurricular activities like?
  - Enquire if the group regularly organises events such as lunches, dinners, or perhaps even laboratory retreats
  - View the university or institution as a whole and see if they offer anything that is very appealing with respect to socialising, sport etc.

## Making an application

Applications for graduate courses, including PhDs, are often made directly to universities or institutions themselves, which are then processed by their own respective departments for the particular course or project concerned. Though, for Master's programmes a central application process is in the pipeline. In most cases, you will be asked to complete a form (usually online) and enter details regarding your academic achievements to date, relevant work experience, extracurricular activities, as well as append a copy of your most recent academic transcript, current curriculum vitae (CV) and a 'personal statement'. Academic references from at least two referees are also usually required, which may in some cases need to be sent or uploaded separately from your own application by your referees.

Some universities or individual research groups may prefer to conduct the application process differently, following a procedure that is similar but nonetheless separate from the main graduate application thread. On this informal basis, you may be asked to complete a smaller application form instead, one that specifically restricts the amount of detail you can enter, including a cover letter and a current CV. Furthermore, you may be expected to simply list the names and email addresses of up to three academic referees, who will then be contacted by the programme administrator themselves. Once the award of a place has been given, the chosen candidate will then be advised to complete and submit a detailed application; though, this will only be treated as a formality rather than an actual application *per se*.

Before you make an application, it's important to familiarise yourself with the admissions process that is being used by the research department you wish to apply to, in particular, whether applications are expected to be made using the main graduate application form (either online or less commonly on paper) or by another informal approach. It goes without saying that deadlines should be carefully noted, not least because a distinction is sometimes drawn between submission of the main application form and receipt of individual academic references, which in the latter case may require you to be in regular contact with your referees.

Turning to some of the specifics of any given application, some components will hold more weight than others and sufficient time and care should be taken in preparing them. The personal statement comes first as it is arguably the most important component, serving to vocalise your desire and justification for wanting to pursue a PhD, which gives it more reason to be scrutinised heavily. Here, you should start by following the guidelines that are typically set out by universities on their webpages, which specifies the point of a personal statement and what assessors will be looking for. The example guidelines listed in Box 2.2 are taken from the University of Oxford's

**Box 2.2** Example components of a PhD personal statement

The personal statement should be a maximum of one page in English and should focus on your interest in, and experience of this research field (rather than personal achievements, interests and aspirations).
This will be assessed for:

- your reasons for applying
- evidence of motivation for and understanding of the proposed area of study
- the ability to present a reasoned case in English
- commitment to the subject, beyond the requirements of the degree course
- preliminary knowledge of research techniques
- capacity for sustained and intense work
- reasoning ability
- ability to absorb new ideas, often presented abstractly, at a rapid pace.

Infection and Immunity Course; and are largely representative of what is expected from any PhD personal statement.

Take the time to write enough drafts while getting feedback from your current supervisor or your academic peers. Indeed, it helps if you have a supervisor on hand to oversee your application, and to consult them for advice on the relevant details. Never use a generic cover letter or personal statement for multiple PhD applications, tailor them carefully for each application you make or else you're unlikely to survive the shortlisting stage.

Your current CV should serve a basic run-down of all your academic and personal achievements to date. In addition, be sure to include all your research experiences that are relevant to the project you are applying for.

## Interviews

If offered an interview, this signals your application is under serious consideration. Unlike undergraduate interviews, which may be offered to many more candidates than there are places, interviews for PhDs are focused on a select few serious candidates. While you should draw confidence from this, now is not the time for complacency: preparation is paramount. Ensure you're clear on what the project is about; the relevant background and existing work in the field (including key publications); your prospective supervisor and their key publications. You must be familiar with and ready to articulate any aspect of your own CV and achievements, including how they are relevant to your career and proposed research.

Interviews vary in their style and formality. They range from an informal conversation with a potential supervisor or small group of two or three people, to a full panel of senior academics; both have their own set of opportunities and challenges. An informal meeting is no less of an interview, be ready to respond to cues and show you've done your homework. With a rapport established, you'll have the flexibility to shape the interview. Be inquisitive but don't avoid talking about yourself where necessary. Remember, your supervisor wants to know whether you'll get on over the next 3 years or more, so let your personality show. Light humour (if well placed) can strengthen your cause. As always, be prepared for the odd query on maths, science, the Big Bang and so on; see later in this chapter for the top 10 questions to be ready to answer and ask.

More formal interview panels, typically encountered during grant or stipend applications, will require inside-out knowledge of the project; often significant preliminary results (and discussion thereof); a formal presentation (e.g. PowerPoint) and a CV and list of personal achievements. It's not uncommon to be required to bring or show examples of your written work too. You'll be fielding questions from interviewers of varying backgrounds, potentially including patient or lay panel members who bring a non-scientific perspective to the (largely public funded) medical science field. Be polite, respectful and ensure you have the necessary documents, directions and dress code information to hand; you might look good in a three-piece suit but will be a tad overdressed for a post-interview tour of the animal facility. Irrespective of the specific interview context, panellists are looking for you to demonstrate a common set of qualities: someone who is enthusiastic and knowledgeable about the proposed work; can demonstrate the right skills and background leading up to the project; has a good understanding of the relevant and likely stages in achieving the proposed objective(s), and who can communicate well with others.

## How to fund one

Funding your PhD is one of the most important issues you and your supervisor must navigate. Levels of funding vary depending on a range of factors, including the type of PhD programme and your career stage. The three key components of your funding are tuition fees, student maintenance (stipend or salary) and the consumables budget that pays for your experiments, reagents and so on. If you're lucky, the funding for these will be organised for you, most likely as part of a 'ready to go' project. If you're not in this boat: read on.

Whatever your track, discuss which funding sources are most suitable with your potential supervisor well in advance. Unless funding is already provided on an existing grant or one specifically awarded for the project, you'll likely be making applications prior to starting the project. For science track candidates, your objective will be to attain all or part of your funding from the following: your department (e.g. existing grants), institution (e.g. university scholarships), research body (e.g. Medical Research Council (MRC), Wellcome Trust) or charity (e.g. CRUK, BHF). A typical consumables budget can reach around £10 000 per year, while a competitive fixed student-level stipend will reach £12 000–17 000 per year. Note that the increasing prevalence of '1 + 3' programmes can mitigate the need for searching for funding, by guaranteeing you a PhD stipend and budget while still allowing flexibility on your PhD project. The 'Gateway to Research'[1] online portal is a powerful tool to examine existing grants and research projects.

For those on a clinical track, your options are a little broader. Those applying for MB-PhD programmes or for a Clinical Research Fellowship are guaranteed funding as part of the programme. ACFs may serve as an initial financial supplement to a PhD, though this requires prior organising and you'll still need to secure further funding as detailed in Box 2.3. MB-PhD programmes pay the typical student stipend; Clinical Research Fellowships vary depending on your career stage and NHS salary but can reach or exceed £40 000–50 000 per year. Clinical research fellows will be expected to maintain clinical commitments such as covering clinical sessions or regularly being on call. As a final option for clinicians (or wealthy non-clinicians), depending on your career stage you might be able to self-fund your PhD, ordinarily by supplementing it with clinical locuming or other work. While this is not encouraged as a long-term strategy, it can act as a temporary 'bridging' solution while waiting for other more robust funding to begin. Most PhD schedules are flexible enough to allow some ad hoc clinical work or alternatively you can work evenings or weekends. However, note that at certain institutions this may not be permissible and full funding arrangements will be expected prior to starting a PhD project. Even if you are able to embark without all your funding allocated, PhD research is intense and demands a level of sustained concentration; clinical commitments can – and often do – interfere.

---

**Box 2.3** Example list of major funding bodies for Clinical Research Fellowships

- MRC, also in collaboration with specific institutions, for example, Wellcome, Francis Crick.
- Royal Colleges.
- Major Medical Research Charities: Wellcome Trust, Cancer Research UK, British Heart Foundation.
- Specific Research Charities: Dunhill Trust, SPARKS, Kidney Research UK, or other members of the Association for Medical Research Charities (AMRC).

---

**Box 2.4** Key components of a grant application

- Personal details of yourself (your CV) and your supervisor (including a personal statement by you and one regarding your suitability from your supervisor, that is relevant to the project in question).
- Your supervisor's key publications and perhaps their CV.
- The project proposal, that is, what are you going to do/trying to achieve (usually at least 1000 words, including as many relevant preliminary results as possible) in scientific language, and sometimes with an additional summary in lay terms.
- Financial details of the funding (including your salary component and each aspect of the equipment and consumables required/claimed for).
- Other supporting documents such as a statement from the head of the department or other departments, for example finance, research services.

---

Writing a grant application will test a range of important skills including your patience, writing, planning and analytic skills – see Box 2.4 for further details. If you're unsure of your suitability for a PhD, by the end of this process you'll know the answer. Several books and articles exist on writing a successful application. Here we shall cover this process briefly. As an early or prospective PhD student, having convincing preliminary results can make the difference between a successful and unsuccessful application. This data might be generated during a BSc or MSc/Res research project, or as part of the first year of your PhD. Members of your research group, might have additional data (published or unpublished) that can support your proposal.

Financial details must be calculated using the online platform *InfoEd*. This takes into account institutional and administrative costs of facilities and services, as well as validating any salary claims. Your university research office may be required to do this for you; if not, you may need training in this electronic system if you're going to be making applications on a regular basis. Most grant awarding bodies require sign off from your own institution before accepting the application; it's therefore prudent to build an understanding with the finance officers/managers in your department or institution in advance to ensure efficient communication.

*Top tips*

Here are 10 interview questions you should be prepared to answer:

1. Why are you doing a PhD and how do you see your career progressing beyond this?
2. What would a successful PhD look like to you?
3. What skills and experience can you bring to this PhD?
4. What (clinical) applications can you see as an outcome of this project?
5. What was your favourite subject at school (i.e. not medicine-related!) and why?
6. What would you have been interested in doing if not science?
7. Related to academic achievement (especially with non-clinical supervisors):
   o What prizes have you gained and for what subjects?
   o What was your academic ranking in your undergraduate degree (e.g. BSc)?
8. What is your 'style' of research and what would expect from a supervisor?
9. Can you describe how you first got interested in research?
10. Tell us about a previous research project – what techniques/approaches did you use and what were your findings?

Here are 10 interview questions you should be prepared to ask.

1. Is the project already funded for the duration?
2. What other funding processes would/might I need to undertake?
3. Who else would help to 'supervise' me first-hand, for example, post-doctoral research fellows, senior technicians?
   o Would it be possible to meet these members of the team before making an application?
4. Who might be the second supervisor?
5. Are all the scientific and technical facilities required (anticipated) to be available at the home institution?
   o Does my supervisor have pre-existing collaborative links with these teams/departments?
6. What additional training courses might I expect to attend and are they available at the home institution?
7. What other training facilities, for example, graduate courses, are available to enrich the overall educational programme?
8. Are there potential international collaborative opportunities to utilise during this PhD?
9. Are students encouraged to publish their work?
10. Are students encouraged to present their work, including internationally?

## Reference

1. Research Councils UK. Gateway to Research, available at: http://gtr.rcuk. ac.uk/(accessed 8 December, 2016).

## Further reading

1. Funston, G. Cerra, C., Kirkham, D., Doherty, G., O'Neill, P. The road to a clinical academic career. BMJ Careers 2015. http://careers.bmj.com/careers/advice/The_road_to_a_clinical_academic_career (accessed 8 December, 2016).
2. Find A PhD, available online https://www.findaphd.com/search/(accessed 8 December, 2016).
3. Williams, K., Bethell, E., Lawton, J., Parfitt-Brown, C., Richardson, M., Victoria, R. Planning Your PhD – Pocket Study Skills. Palgrave-Macmillan 2010.
4. Barnett-Vanes, A., Ho, G., Cox, TM. Clinician-scientist MB/PhD training in the UK: a nationwide survey of medical school policy. BMJ Open. 2015 30; 5(12):e009852.

# Chapter 3   **Anatomy of a PhD: Where you fit in the academic world**

*Laura Lambert[1] and John Tregoning[2]*

[1] Post-doctoral researcher, Imperial College London, UK
[2] Senior Lecturer, Imperial College London, UK

## Background: Welcome to the new you

The basics: we wrote this from two perspectives, one of us is a senior lecturer (John) who started their PhD last century, but still thinks he has something useful to say (a defining feature of academics!); the other (Laura) is a millennial who recently completed her PhD. Throughout this chapter, we'll speak for ourselves, each other and occasionally as one.

John: It's safe to assume that on starting your PhD you have more of an idea about academia than I did at an equivalent point. However, in order to cover everything, I am going to target this chapter at the me aged 22, who undertook a PhD as a filler till something else better came along (near two decades later, and I am still waiting). If you are as ill-prepared as I was, a guide to who all these lab people are, what they do and where you fit in should be of value. And when they (or you) invent time-travel, I can send this chapter back to myself and avoid a few of my freshman gaffes.

Laura: If someone had told the 15-year-old me that 6 years down the line I would begin a PhD, I would have pictured my future self as a studious and achingly intelligent woman: prone to witty dinner party badinage, intimidatingly well organised; far too on top of life to be bothered by trivialities. The truth is, there is no new 'you'; just a new challenge. If you have successfully navigated your academic life so far – including securing a PhD – while being the kind of person often found on a sofa in a onesie, streaming cat videos, you probably aren't going to change now. Either way, the point here is to not be phased by anyone else's 'PhD student persona' (I am the owner of multiple onesies) and instead focus on yourself. Most of my peers from my undergraduate days are earning eye-watering salaries as lawyers and bankers in the

*How to Complete a PhD in the Medical and Clinical Sciences*,
First Edition. Edited by Ashton Barnett-Vanes and Rachel Allen.
© 2018 John Wiley & Sons Ltd. Published 2018 by John Wiley & Sons Ltd.

City, yet it has pleasantly surprised me that at social gatherings it is my work that garners the most interest. For these situations, it's useful to have an upbeat and shall we say creative layman's summary of your research on standby. For example, my work on neonatal lung infections translates to 'I basically save babies'. Wholly inaccurate of course, but on a serious note, anything that piques scientific interest (or gets them to pay the dinner bill) can only be a good thing.

## You are here: PhD research versus undergraduate studies

*John*: If you take one lesson away from reading this chapter let it be: 'Doing a PhD is nothing like being an undergraduate'. Yes, 'you're still a student', as your friends who have gone on to do other more lucrative but less interesting jobs will tell you; yes, it's still in the ivory towers/concrete blockwork of an academic institution; yes, it's still possible to (occasionally) come in after 10 am; but otherwise it's a completely different experience. You're now entering a world where having represented the university at ping pong and being chair of the underwater basket-weaving society counts for nothing.

*Laura*: The key thing about being a PhD student is that the 'student' title is a misnomer. It is basically a job, albeit one with a very relaxed dress code.

*John*: In fact, it's worth highlighting at this point that there are two parts to universities. There is the side of the university that belongs to the undergrads, made up of the bar, lecture theatre, pub, practical-lab and night club. The interactions of undergraduates with academics are limited to termly meetings with a personal tutor, who often has to look up your name to remember who you are, lectures, and tutorials that you are ill-prepared for. There is then the other university, the one you have now entered: the research university. This is the world of the PhD, post-doc, Principle Investigator (PI), RA, and Professor. On the whole, the two universities don't mix, indeed the best time of year in the research university is the long summer vacation when all the undergrads have gone home and there is peace, quiet and no teaching.

*Laura*: Transitioning from the structured lecture/lab timetables, assignment hand-ins and specified term dates of an undergraduate degree to managing your own time and project during a PhD definitely requires a lot more of that dreaded 'self-motivation'. This isn't quite as daunting as it sounds. There are still deadlines to keep to: writing transfer reports, preparing presentations for lab meetings and making posters for conferences, which force you to keep yourself in check. In a similar vein, one of the most important differences between PhD and undergraduate is that your project is – by definition – a novel piece of work, and therefore somewhat of an unpredictable and untamed beast. No matter how many Gantt charts you churn out, and how detailed your research proposal, it will probably run off on a tangent as untamed beasts are wont to do. To me, this is the most exciting aspect of PhD research: at undergraduate level, you learn knowledge that already exists, while as a doctoral student you get to create new knowledge, which with a bit of luck will one day end up in the former's text book.

## Lab types: A field guide

What follows is a broad generalisation of the different roles, which will hopefully give you some idea of who the people around you are; but clearly, everyone is different, all labs are structured in different ways and what works in a UK immunology lab may not be the case in a Danish neuroscience department. The key is to be nice to everyone you meet; primarily because it's the right thing to do but also because occasionally you'll need someone to sort out your bursary, explain flow cytometry or free you from a toilet with a broken door handle.

### The student (you)

There is no 'standard issue' variety of PhD student. Most labs contain a motley crew of ages and nationalities. From bright-eyed recent graduates to part-time student 'veterans', labs are a diverse place. First and foremost, a PhD is an apprenticeship in science. Students are often seen as a source of youthful energy in the lab, and what they lack in experience they make up for in enthusiasm (initially). Students are also a constant source of wonder for more senior members of the team – 'you would not believe what they did this time'. Depending on the lab, you will be perceived as a cheap pair of hands, a costly obligation, a chance to pass on learning to the next generation or all three at the same time. Projects normally start as being quite directed to enable you to learn the trade, but hopefully end up with the opportunity to design and execute your own experiments.

*John*: Over the course of the PhD, in addition to learning science you will be expected to learn to be an adult human being, take responsibility for your future, gain core employability skills and how to make a decent cup of tea for your supervisor (worth a try).

### Technicians

*John*: These break down into two very broad categories, lab 'techs' and research techs. Lab techs are the people who make labs function via a range of critical tasks like ordering supplies, preparing media and re-stocking the consumables. Joining a lab with a good lab tech will save you a lot of time that can then be spent on research (or, if you are one of my students, looking at pictures of dogs with interesting haircuts). Research techs (sometimes called research assistants – 'RAs') are involved in running core assays. RT/RAs have great experimental expertise and are the go to people for troubleshooting assays when things go wrong. There is another group of technicians who run specific bits of equipment – flow cytometers, histology, microscopes, diamond light sources and so on. Highly specialised and very focused, they don't like you breaking (or even using) their equipment and will let you know very quickly how and where you have broken their equipment.

*Laura*: Lab technicians know where everything is and have the coveted golden touch when it comes to the protocols that no one else can get to work. Some believe they are magical. Stay on their good side.

## Support staff

The most important, but least thanked people in the university. These are the accountants, lab managers, PhD programme directors, animal handlers, health and safety inspectors and so on. Universities are big, complex organisations, often located in ancient buildings designed for an entirely different purpose. Academics are brilliant (sometimes) but impractical (often) egomaniacs (always) and if things were left to them the whole organisation would collapse. To ensure the institution gets from day-to-day, there is a large supporting cast from the woman who knows how to get you an R2D2 (or BB-8) transistor to the man who sells cups of tea.

## Post-docs

Once upon a time, the academic job structure went PhD-Post-doc; Post-doc-lecturer. Post-docs are the next step in the academic career path. Post-docs have learned how to be a scientist during their PhD and are now applying these skills to a range of problems, with less supervision and more independence. There can be a high turnover rate, but each new researcher brings fresh protocols, wisdom and experience from their previous projects.

*Laura*: However, there is a tension in being a post-doc. They are trying to balance their own needs, the boss's needs and the project's needs. This can occasionally bubble over when you, as a youthful but naïve PhD student, demand their time to teach you how to do an ELISA (for the nth time): tread carefully!

## PIs (principle investigators)
### Junior PIs (lecturers/associate professors)

A fragile beast. They are either trying to get their first tenured (permanent contract) track position, have just got their first tenured track position or are trying to justify why they should keep their tenure track position.

In new/small groups a lot of the PI's hopes depend on the quality of your PhD data. As such, you may experience intense micromanagement – since the PI is no longer able to be lab active, their experiments are vicariously performed through you: 'Have you counted those cytospins yet?', 'Where is the data from the 6-week-long experiment you only started yesterday?'. Despite this being their first time in the role, they are still your boss and need your support and reassurance.

### Senior PIs (Professors)

Last engaged in labwork when mouth pipetting and smoking in the lab were still *en vogue*. Usually brilliant, very experienced, often remote. Professors tend to have large groups and their attention will be diluted between these members as well as their university administrative duties and external facing work. The caricature in 'piled higher and deeper'[1] isn't a million miles off. There is a special subset called Emeritus Professors, who are retired from all the admin and teaching and can now focus their time on finding science fascinating.

In summary, laboratories are large complex organisations, with a bunch of different people who make the research go forwards. Your interactions with the different people in your lab, will define your PhD experience.

### A note on advanced academic-ology

Just to add confusion, PIs have ranks, which will have various titles according to local tradition. In the UK, it goes Lecturer–Senior Lecturer–Reader–Professor, in the USA it goes Assistant Professor–Associate Professor–Professor and Wikipedia can fill in the gaps in local knowledge for elsewhere. These ranks have little impact on the actual day-to-day job of the PI but they are important to the people who hold them.

### It's tricky: The student-supervisor interaction

*John*: The key relationship for the next three years is between you and your supervisor. The supervisor-student relationship is complex. Good or bad, this relationship will shape the entire course of your PhD (and your future life in science). There are tales of a supervisor's influence being so strong that the student found themselves stirring tea in the same way as their ex-boss. That's probably apocryphal, but I do occasionally catch myself sitting in a certain way during meetings and seeing my post-doc supervisor in myself. As both a parent and a supervisor, there are certain similarities in the relationship, though I tend to micromanage my children more and swear in front of them less.

In science PhDs, nine times out of ten, the initiator of the project is the supervisor and so the idea and an awful lot of emotional investment have been put into it by them. For clinical PhDs, the project may have been initiated together with, or even by, the student, which will slightly change the dynamic. In arts PhDs – well let's just not go there… Either way, at the start the supervisor will know more than you about the subject matter, the techniques, scientific method, the way to write and so on. The balance of scientific knowledge will change over the course of the PhD and at some point, you will be the expert in the microfluidics of drosophila lungs or whatever highly niche subject you are working on. Even then, the supervisor will have more experience of some of the other skills, like science writing, job hunting, writing you a reference and regardless, will need to sign off on most of the above. Ultimately, you should always aim for the relationship to be one of mutual respect.

*Laura*: From the student perspective, the role of the supervisor can swing wildly between boss, friend, nanny, amanuensis, hero and nemesis from one day to the next. As with any relationship, patience is key, as is understanding that your supervisor is likely to have other students or colleagues demanding their time and energy. Don't be the whiny youngest child. On the other hand, compared to bosses in most other job sectors, supervisors are 'in charge' of relatively few people and this is what makes the relationship such a unique one. You should therefore expect to see and interact with your supervisor on a regular basis – no excuses. Emotional involvement in the project is where issues can and do occur. At some point, mid-PhD, I started getting a sort of vague gut feeling as to whether an experiment was going to give any useful results – a kind of maternal instinct borne out of so many hours spent in the lab with my 'baby' (the project – keep up). Of course, this instinct is never infallible, but on balance I found it to be quite a solid indicator of which experimental path to pursue. Since the supervisor spends far less time personally conducting the experiments and thus lacks this particular radar, it can be difficult to convince them that *The Instinct* is not merely laziness, but it is best to remain constructive and strategic. Supervisors are well placed to get to know your particular strengths, weaknesses and personality quirks, and thus can be a great source of career guidance and job references in the future. If in doubt, ride it out, it's only 3 years…

See Chapter 6 for further details on dealing with supervisor problems.

## Check out my massive organogram

*John*: In theory, a university is more than the sum of its individual research groups, but then again organising academics is routinely described as herding cats. There is a structure and the group you are in will slot into this somewhere. Why should this matter to you? Firstly, departments have bigger budgets than groups and so can throw better parties. Secondly, there is often department level funding that may cover your trips to conferences. Thirdly, there will be people working on similar areas who can help you with your research. Finally, did I mention the parties?

Again, it's hard not to generalise and you'll need to find out what the local situation is (look out for departmental organisational charts, see Figure 3.1). Once upon a time it was simple, there was a department, the head of which was the chair (the only Professor in the department) and everyone else had to do what the Professor said. Nowadays the structure can be much more diffuse. A common structure is: group (you + your supervisor + whoever else works for them), section (a vague collective of academics working in a similar field), department (same as section, but more people and a wider scope of study) and faculty (a range of departments competing and collaborating). At the most basic, these structures are purely administrative, pooling resources, particularly the back-office functions such as finances, grants management, tech support and so on. But when they work well, they are groupings of like minded academics, working on a similar field to a common purpose, with a mutual support network.

Within these structures, the most important and relevant interactions for you will be the people who occupy the same lab space. This will normally be your group, but will often include one or two other groups who for economies of scale have been squeezed into the same space or share equipment. This is normally good news – giving you a wider circle of similar level people to get ideas, support and steal reagents from. But, occasionally the lab heads will fall out leading to frosty relations that trickle down to lab members. Be considerate to those around you and discover the art of being recognised for any good corporate citizenship: there's no point in cleaning the lab if no one notices!

*Laura*: When not in the lab, you'll probably be housed in an office or desk area with your fellow students, who may or may not be in the same research field. The objective of this is to allow for helpful discussions and sharing of ideas between those at similar stages in their career; a 'cross-pollination' between different fields if you will. My over-riding memories of our infamous 'PhD Office' involve mostly the helpful discussions around weekend plans, the sharing of internet memes, and the gossip about who was currently engaging in 'cross-pollination' with each other.

## Other dull, but important stuff

### Graduate school

*John*: The graduate school exists to oversee your non-lab based personal development. Once seen as solely for tapping up for loan extensions, overseas trips, travel grants and providing courses with free biscuits. However, as the

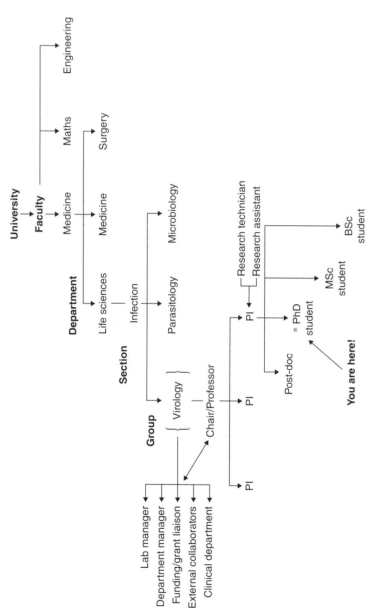

**Figure 3.1** University hierarchy

vast majority of scientific PhD graduates will go into non-academic roles after graduation (see Chapter 10 for more on graduate outcomes), graduate schools now place much greater emphasis in PhD training on developing transferable skills and experience to enhance future employability.

*Laura*: Most of my interaction with the graduate school was one-sided in the form of emails from it reminding me that – in order to fulfil the criteria to be awarded my degree – I was to attend various personal development courses. There were quite a few to choose from ranging from 'How to Present a Poster' to the slightly alarmingly-titled 'Assertiveness'. While I grumbled about how much precious lab time these courses stole (reality: half a day), I found that most were worth it, and attending them earlier in your PhD rather than leaving it until the hectic final few months is definitely advised. In particular, residential courses can be a great chance to enjoy a little institution-sponsored largesse, while forming new friendships and connections with those from parts of the university you might otherwise never meet.

### Part-time and full-time

*John*: While most PhD students will be full-time with a stipend, student card and a terrible haircut; others will be doing a PhD part-time in addition to doing a job – normally on the same subject. In practice, there is not much difference, but occasionally the pressures of the job for a part-time student can get in the way of delivering on their research. This is a challenging balance to strike and it's important you recognise the checkpoints and timelines expected of a part-time PhD should you elect for this route.

### Conclusion

*Laura*: My final piece of advice is a classic for good reasons: try to keep everything in perspective. Don't be intimidated by the egos or extremes of personality types you may encounter; but appreciate the structure and where you fit in. Don't over-react to one abrupt response from your supervisor and resolve to pack in the whole thing after a week, but do listen calmly to any constructive criticism you may receive. You will soon find yourself showing the next batch of new students the ropes, tutting just like your supervisor when they use up all the ethanol without ordering more, and lo, the Circle of Lab Life begins again.

*John*: Universities are big, complex, arcane organisations with tribal hierarchies, local rules and individual idiosyncrasies. Your priority is to negotiate your interactions, particularly between you and your supervisor, but also between you and anyone else in the lab. Beware, scientists are fickle, gossipy and not great with change, this means that first impressions are really important, you can recover from a bad start but you will create work for yourself. Likewise, don't behave well for your first week only to make a fool of yourself in the pub on the first Friday. Science is small, your field smaller still, and you don't want to be known as 'that person'. The good news is, sooner or later, other new people will join the lab and everyone will forget the time you did that thing, you know, the one we don't mention.

## Reference

1. PhD Comics, website available at www.phdcomics.com (accessed 8 December, 2016).

# Chapter 4 Core techniques, principles and statistics

*Andrew John Walley[1], Kyrillos N Adesina-Georgiadis[2], Adel Benlahrech[3] and Fiona Reid[4]*

[1] Senior Lecturer in Human Genomics, St George's, University of London, UK

[2] Honorary Research Associate, Imperial College London, UK

[3] Post-doctoral researcher, University of Oxford, UK

[4] Senior Lecturer in Statistics, King's College London and St George's, University of London, UK

## Genomics

Understanding of the umbrella term 'Omics' has become important for anyone working in the medical and clinical sciences. This is due to the many recent advances in medicine using these technologies, as well as the future promise they hold. In its simplest definition, Omics is the study of all areas of scientific interest that are described by terms with the suffix –ome (see Table 4.1 for examples).

At present, those omics techniques of most interest to PhD students will be those widely used for analysing nucleic acids (DNA and RNA) and proteins.

### Nucleic acids

Over the last 15 years, two major technological advances have been responsible for the rapid progress made in analysing nucleic acids with respect to health and disease. The first was the development of oligonucleotide arrays, which allowed researchers to measure the levels of all the mRNA in a biological sample, or to type very large numbers of genetic markers across the whole genome. The second was the development of high-throughput, massively parallel, next generation sequencing (NGS). The major companies in these fields are Affymetrix Inc. (Arrays) and Illumina Inc. (Arrays and NGS).

### *Oligonucleotide arrays*

Gene expression arrays work on the principle of immobilising single-stranded DNA molecules of known sequence (usually short oligonucleotides) on a solid support, hybridising them with single-stranded nucleic acid

*How to Complete a PhD in the Medical and Clinical Sciences*,
First Edition. Edited by Ashton Barnett-Vanes and Rachel Allen.

**Table 4.1** Examples of –omes and their biological object

| -Ome | Biological Object |
|---|---|
| Genome | DNA |
| Exome | Coding DNA (exons)* |
| Transcriptome | RNA |
| Proteome | Protein |
| Epigenome | Epigenetic signals[†] |
| Metabolome | Metabolites |
| Regulome | Regulatory Molecules |
| Lipidome | Lipids |
| Microbiome | Microorganisms[‡] |
| Connectome | Brain Connections |
| Interactome | Protein Interactions |
| Exposome | Environmental exposures |

* The exome can refer to just the coding DNA within all of the genes, to the full set of exons within genes (some of which will be non-coding) or to the complete set of all the gene sequences (including all the regulatory sequences such as promoters).
[†] This includes DNA methylation, histone modifications and other signals.
[‡] This refers to the set of bacterial microorganisms found in a specific environmental niche or location. The fungal microbiome is often referred to separately and the viral microbiome is often referred to as the virome.

(DNA/RNA) sample labelled with a fluorescent dye and then detecting the double-stranded molecules using a scanner. The amount of signal from the label is directly proportional to the amount of labelled nucleic acid that has hybridised. For an RNA sample, this gives a measure of relative gene expression within the sample. To detect gene transcripts, each one is represented on an array by multiple sequences to ensure correct detection. Such arrays can be designed to detect expression of different splice variants. By comparing housekeeping gene expression between samples in the same experiment, it is possible to normalise the data to allow comparisons across samples. It should be noted that gene expression array experiments are not usually considered reproducible enough to allow simple comparison across experiments carried out at different times and in different laboratories. Standardisation of the reporting of experimental protocols, such as MiAME (Minimum information about a microarray experiment), does not compensate for this fundamental problem in comparing experimental results from different studies.

Array technology has allowed the characterisation of gene expression in a wide range of tissues, developmental states and diseases in both humans and animal models. Most strikingly, the use of gene expression arrays introduced the concept of gene profiling to characterise cancers and the idea that single cancers, such as breast cancer, are in fact a group of phenotypically similar cancers that can be distinguished by their gene profiles.

Genetic marker arrays work on a similar principle in the first stage of the assay. The immobilised oligonucleotide is hybridised to unlabelled genomic DNA. In the Illumina assay, the oligonucleotide sequence hybridises adjacent to the single nucleotide polymorphism (SNP) that is to be genotyped. The sequence is extended by a single base using a fluorescently labelled dideoxy-nucleotide. For single nucleotide polymorphisms, there are two possible bases that can be added: the wild-type (wt) and the variant (var), and each is labelled with a different dye. The use of dideoxynucleotide bases prevents any further extension of the double-stranded DNA so the fluorescent signal can be measured. The signal will be all one colour, all the other or a mixture of both (corresponding to the three possible genotypes: wt/wt, var/var and wt/var). The use of arrays allows the genotyping of hundreds of thousands of SNPs simultaneously for a single sample and the rapid genotyping of thousands of samples. The end result has been hundreds of Genome Wide Association Studies (GWAS) for common diseases, identifying many new genes and genomic loci previously unknown to be involved in the pathogenesis of diseases affecting millions of people worldwide.

### Next generation sequencing

At the start of the millennium, the first draft human genome sequence took three years to complete and cost over £100 000 000. At the time of writing, a single genome sequence can be generated in less than a day at a cost of less than £1000, purely due to advances in technology. Illumina Inc. have been at the forefront of developing low-cost, high-throughput, genome sequencing and their platform has proved to be extremely adaptable to other fields of interest within genomics (see Table 4.2 for specific examples).

The Illumina sequencing assay utilises two core techniques: isothermal bridge amplification and sequencing by synthesis. In essence, isothermal bridge amplification is a method by which small, isolated, patches are created across the whole surface of an oligonucleotide array. In each patch are many copies of one short (<500 bases) unknown genomic sequence. Sequencing by synthesis then occurs by the sequential addition of fluorescently labelled bases one at a time, with a scanner recording the fluorescent signal from each patch after each base is added. By recording the signals, these can be translated into a sequence and this is recorded for millions of these patches. Sophisticated software then processes the raw data and aligns the short sequences into a form that is usable in downstream analysis.

The flexibility of this process comes from the fact that the short DNA sequences for sequencing can be derived from any experiment you can think of. They might be cDNA derived from an mRNA sample, they could be bisulfite-modified DNA to determine the presence of 5-methyl cytosine, they could be DNA protected from enzymatic digestion by transcription factors bound to it or by specific chromatin conformations.

**Table 4.2** Examples of methods used to analyse specific genomic targets using NGS technologies

| Analysis Target | Method | Full Name |
|---|---|---|
| DNA | DNA-Seq | DNA sequencing |
|  | WGS | Whole genome sequencing |
|  | Exome-Seq | Exome (all coding regions) sequencing |
| RNA | Total RNA-Seq | RNA Sequencing of all RNA in a sample |
|  | mRNA-Seq | Transcriptome sequencing |
|  | smallRNA-Seq | Small RNA targeted sequencing |
| DNA Methylation | Bis-Seq | Bisulfite modified DNA sequencing |
|  | MeDIP-Seq | Methylated DNA immunoprecipitation sequencing |
|  | RRB-Seq | Reduced representation bisulfite sequencing |
| Transcription factor binding sites | ChIP-Seq | Chromatin immunoprecipitation sequencing |
| Regulatory elements | FAIRE-Seq | Formaldehyde-assisted isolation of regulatory elements |
| Chromatin conformation | 3C | Chromatin conformation capture |
|  | 4C | Chromatin conformation capture circular |
|  | 5C | Chromatin conformation capture carbon copy |
|  | ChIA-Pet | Chromatin interaction analysis by paired-end tag sequencing |

**Proteins**

Protein Omics techniques are aimed at characterising all the proteins present in a biological sample. Electrophoretic techniques have been around for a long time that allow the visualisation of a complex mixture of proteins. While one-dimensional electrophoresis can successfully separate mixtures of proteins, the use of a second dimension for separation greatly increases the resolving power of this method. Typically, two-dimensional-electrophoresis separates proteins in the first dimension on the basis of their isoelectric point (pI) and in the second dimension on the basis of their mass. This allows the identification of differences in complex mixtures of proteins, even down to single amino acid changes due to a disease-causing mutation. However, the resolving power of this technique is relatively limited and identification of specific proteins can be very difficult.

High-Performance Liquid Chromatography (HPLC) is a highly flexible method for separating out components of a mixture of biomolecules. Essentially, the mixture of interest is added to a flow of solvent (mobile phase) that carries it through a column packed with a filtering material (stationary phase). The material flowing out from the column is then passed through a detector and aliquots containing detected material are collected for further analysis. The specific attributes of the stationary phase allow the filtering of the protein mixture on the basis of a number of characteristics depending on the column material chosen. Separation is often carried out by physical size, charge or hydrophobicity. Columns can also be created that utilise immobilised antibodies to remove specific proteins or proteins with specific domains. HPLC is routinely used in the analysis of biological samples of unknown characteristics, as well as in diagnostics where the behaviour of a specific protein is well characterised and easily measured. The main disadvantage of HPLC is that it can only separate out proteins where they differ significantly in how they interact with the stationary phase.

Mass spectrometry has become the method of choice for proteomics because it is highly accurate and reproducible. There are many different approaches currently used but one of the most popular is peptide analysis using MALDI-TOF. Rather than try to analyse very large protein molecules directly, protein mixtures are digested using proteases, such as trypsin, and the resulting mix of smaller peptides is analysed. MALDI-TOF MS, or matrix assisted desorption ionisation time-of-flight mass spectrometry, is a commonly used method for both peptide and small oligonucleotide analysis. A sample of the peptide mixture is spotted onto an ordered array, placed at one end of a vacuum tube and then each sample is sequentially vaporised and ionised by a laser. A high voltage difference is then applied between the two ends of the tube and the time it takes the ionised molecules to reach the opposite end of the tube and be detected is directly proportional to their mass and charge. The generated profile can then be compared to known sets of fragments generated by proteolytic digestion and known proteins identified and subtracted, leaving unknown peaks to be identified. Given the very large number of fragments that can be generated by digestion of a biological sample, HPLC is routinely used to separate the complex mixture into a set of samples with a smaller range of fragments in each one that can then be analysed by MS.

## Conclusion

Omics techniques are already being used in the clinic, with cancer profiling in wide usage for breast cancer and being pushed heavily for other cancers. Next generation sequencing of rare monogenic diseases is on the brink of routine clinical usage, with clear benefits in its application already demonstrated in national genetic centres across the world. Without doubt, Omics techniques are here to stay and will become ever more common in PhD student projects.

## Metabolomics

Recent scientific effort within biomedical research has extensively involved molecular characterisation of disease phenotypes. This has led to a drive for the development of new techniques for the improvement of our understanding of the molecular and cellular alterations underlying disease and how these relate to pathophysiological and toxic events. Defined as the 'quantitative measurement of the dynamic multiparametric metabolic response of living systems to pathophysiological stimuli or genetic modification'[1], metabolomics is concerned with the observation of small molecules within a biological sample. Metabolomics is a 'top-down' systems biology approach and as such can provide a direct picture of cellular activity, health status and the effects of disease, drugs or the environment. It is therefore an ideal tool for the identification of biomarkers and pathways of disease and/or toxicity, stratification of patients into responder groups and the construction of models for diagnostic or regulatory purposes.

Biofluids, such as blood serum or urine, or tissues that have undergone chemical extraction are investigated by analytical techniques, primarily NMR Spectroscopy and Mass spectrometry, the latter normally being coupled to a chemical separation process such as liquid or gas chromatography. Optical spectrometric techniques, such as matrix assisted desorption (MALDI), can also be used for localised analysis. All these techniques provide information on the endogenous and exogenous metabolites present and a metabolic spectrum is generated. These outputs are very data rich, and many times include complicated or noisy data, which is multicollinear and can contain variation from multiple sources, including electronic noise. For the adequate interpretation and comprehension of the signals, visualisation and identification of the main sources of variation, computer pattern recognition and related statistical and computational approaches, collectively known as chemometrics, are employed. The multivariate modelling methods routinely utilised include projection based statistics, which can be unsupervised, such as Principal Component Analysis, or supervised, such as Partial Least Square Regression and its variants[2].

### Metabolomics in a PhD project

Metabolomics can be employed as the sole technology within a PhD, and will usually involve the application of said methods to a novel disease or compound. Within toxicology, the investigation of the metabolism of xenobiotics remains the major focus of metabolomics; while patient stratification through metabolic profiling is the primary concern of disease research. In either case, the project would likely comprise three key stages: sample collection, sample analysis and finally chemometric analysis. Sample collection involves the collection of the target biofluid or tissue, either from an animal model or from humans, although cell/tissue cultures are also used. The PhD student may not directly be involved with this aspect, depending on the involvement of trained animal handlers or clinicians. These samples will then be prepared for analysis by the choice analytical technology. Traditionally a project would focus on utilising one particular platform (be it MS or NMR); however, there is now a trend towards applying both in order to achieve wider metabolome coverage. This analysis stage may also involve the development of new analytical methods, especially in novel compound groups, and this can comprise a large part of analysis time. Finally, once profiling is complete, chemometric analysis should be employed to ascertain the key metabolites of interest and to identify what these metabolites are. Identification of metabolites can involve further targeted experiments for full validation.

## Combination technologies

Finally, various combinations of Omics technologies have been attempted including integration of genomics, transcriptomics, proteomics, localisomics and phenomics using various methods such as the MODEM algorithms and the COBRA method. Metabolomics has also been a part of this and combined studies with data from other Omic technologies have now become common place. Combining metabolic data with genetic data is now well established, and is called metabolic quantities trait mapping (mQTL), whereas combining metabolism with 16s RNA sequencing of the gut-microbiota is now very popular in the investigation of diseases modulated by microflora such as obesity and Irritable Bowel Syndrome.

Metabolomics provides a molecular snapshot of the samples and as such can be described as a functional phenotype. However, it is important to see that as the focus of research moves from genes to transcription factors to enzymes to proteins, the information gathered is increasingly remote to primary regulation. This means that there is an effect gradient between genetic regulation and metabolism, resulting in associations that are hard to classify depending on the divergence of final outcome from the causal gene. Correlating metabolic profile data with data from other types of analyses is perhaps the only way of correctly mapping primary aberrations in the DNA with actual downstream events.

## Common pitfalls

1. *Not understanding the technology employed*
   While in many fields of science much of the research instruments can be used as 'black boxes', it is essential for metabonomic research that the user understands the theory of the analytical techniques. Understanding why

the intensity MS signal depends on the ability of the metabolite to ionise not on the amount present, for example, is crucial for the correct conclusions to be reached.

2. *Not understanding the computational bits*
   Metabolomics depends on many different computational methods for data analysis. While using command line stats packages such as R or Python can be daunting, and require high levels of computer literacy, being able to confidently manipulate the data is absolutely essential.

3. *Metabolite identification*
   A common scenario with a metabonomic analysis is discovering a highly significant metabolite, but not knowing what this metabolite actually is. Metabolite identification is not only a skill in of itself, but the identification process can take as long, if not longer, than all the previous steps of the analysis. Much research is in fact published with many significant metabolites listed as 'unassigned'. Care must be taken to ensure that all biomarkers are validated.

4. *Not understanding the biology*
   As a field, metabolomics was pioneered and is still largely practised by analytical chemists. As such, the biological aspects of the system under study can at times be overlooked. However, for completeness it is essential to have a good grasp of the molecular and biological processes, especially if the project is focused on a human disease.

## Flow cytometry

Flow cytometry, which translates to (cyto = cell, metry = measurement using 'flow' mechanics), is a technique through which the properties of cells can be measured. It was first developed and commercialised in 1968 by Walfgang Göhde from the University of Münster. At the time, it was known as pulse cytophotometry and had the capacity to detect two parameters simultaneously. Flow cytometry has come a long way since then and it's now possible to detect up to 20 different parameters concurrently on a single cell. It is widely considered an ideal tool for the analysis of even the rarest cell subsets and their function.

### How does flow cytometry work?

To understand the principles behind flow cytometry, consider the following example:

*Background*: Human blood contains red and white blood cells. The latter are composed of many different types of individual cells, each with a specific function. Some of these cells are termed T cells, which can be identified on the basis of expression of the receptor CD3. T cells can be further subdivided into CD4+ and CD8+ T cells depending on whether they express CD4 or CD8 molecules on their surface.

*Question:* How would you determine the proportions of CD4 and CD8 T cells within your sample?

*Answer:* Flow cytometry can be used to identify the composition of your sample. In this particular example, you would incubate your blood sample with antibodies that specifically bind to CD3, CD4 and CD8 receptors. Each of these antibodies will be conjugated (bound) to a different fluorochrome. These, which are also known as fluorophores, are small molecules that are capable of emitting light of a specific wavelength when excited by a laser. You would then acquire the sample using a flow cytometer that will pass single cells through a laser beam thereby exciting the different fluorochromes. These will in turn emit light with different wavelengths that are picked up by specific detectors. These different 'colours' can then be translated into an electronic signal. You can then process that information using computers that will allow you to identify the composition of your sample (see Figure 4.1).

## Applications

Flow cytometry offers researchers a tool to investigate a range of cells and subsets rapidly. Virtually any tissue can be processed and analysed. However, flow cytometry is not confined to simply measuring expression of cell surface molecules. It occurs in many different formats, which can be adapted for individual applications. A number of cellular functions can be determined by flow cytometry using the following variations.

### *Proliferation assays*

Cellular division can be monitored by labelling cells with a fluorescent dye such as carboxyfluorescein succinimidyl ester (CFSE) or Violet Proliferation Dye (VPD). If a cell divides, the dye will be equally distributed between the daughter cells resulting in half the fluorescence intensity. Transition through the cell cycle can also be visualised using DNA dyes such as 7-Aminoactinomycin D (7AAD) and thymidine analogues such as bromodeoxyuridine (BRDU) or 5-ethynyl-2'-deoxyuridine (EDU).

### *Intracellular cytokine staining (ICS)*

The ability of cells to respond to different stimuli can be visualised by ICS. Principally, cells are incubated in the presence of a protein-transport inhibitor such as monensin or brefeldin-A, so that the produced proteins are prevented from being secreted. Cells are then permeabilised to allow the antibodies to pass through the plasma membrane and access the cytoplasm.

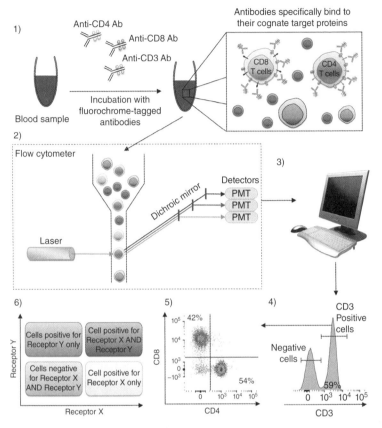

**Figure 4.1** How flow cytometry works

### Phosphoflow
Protein phosphorylation is essential for cell signalling. The phosphorylated states can be identified using antibodies that can distinguish between phosphorylated and non-phosphorylated states of proteins.

### Bead-based immunoassays
It is not only cells that can be analysed by flow cytometry. Soluble proteins within cell culture supernatants, serum, or plasma can be quantified using antibody-coated beads. This technique allows for the quantification of several proteins simultaneously, which gives it an edge over standard enzyme-linked immunosorbent assays (ELISA).

### Prime Flow RNA assays
This is a novel technique that combines mRNA amplification with flow cytometry. This technique allows for the simultaneous measurement of mRNA and protein levels at the single cell level.

### Fluorescence-activated cell sorting (FACS)
In this variation of flow cytometry, cells can be physically separated on the basis of their fluorescent labels. In this case, the flow cytometer would need to be equipped with a sorting unit that applies electrical charges to cell droplets and separates them by electrostatic deflection. The specific cells you 'sort' can then be used in further experiments or analyses.

## Important considerations
### Fluorescence spill-over
Flow cytometry depends on the ability of fluorophores to emit light when excited by lasers. The emission spectra of fluorophores can overlap interfering with data interpretation. This can be corrected through a process known as compensation, which teaches the computer to distinguish between what is a real signal and what is spill-over fluorescence from other fluorochromes picked up by the neighbouring detector.

### True or false
Cells exhibit varying levels of protein expression, discriminating between positive and negative populations is not as easy as it sounds. Isotype controls and fluorescence minus one procedures 'FMO' are used to improve the validity of your positive and negative 'gates'. Remember, these must be specific for each tissue you analyse.

### Live or dead
Cells demonstrate significantly different staining and size properties when they have 'died'. Thus, the use of a 'Live/dead' stain is essential in flow cytometry. In situations where cells can only be analysed the day or week later, 'fixing' reagents composed of paraformaldehyde can be used to preserve the cells' integrity and antibody stains.

### Non-specific staining
Flow cytometry relies on the ability of antibodies to specifically bind to their target proteins. However, antibodies can also attach non-specifically to cells by binding to molecules such as Fc receptors. Isotype controls and Fc blockers such as animal serum or anti-CD16/32 antibodies are often used to address this issue.

### Autofluorescence

Many cells contain molecules that become fluorescent when excited by lasers – alveolar macrophages are one example. These endogenous fluorophores can give rise to false positive results. This can be circumvented by including appropriate negative and positive controls as discussed earlier. A novel technique termed mass cytometry or (CyTOF) removes the issue of autofluorescence altogether by replacing fluorochromes with heavy metal ion tags.

### Sample format

Cells used in flow cytometry can be derived from many different types of specimens. However, they all need to be converted into single cell suspensions prior to running the samples through the flow cytometer. This results in loss of information about the three-dimensional architecture of samples. Similarly, the intracellular localisation of detected proteins is poorly resolved by flow cytometry. Further, enzymatic tissue digestion protocols can degrade the quality of key cell surface protein targets.

### Breakdown

Flow cytometry is powerful but also prone to failure. Machines can get blocked or clogged; lasers can get damaged or deteriorate. Read the whole of the manual for your flow machine, including the section on what to do in the event of a problem. Your institutional flow cytometry technicians are a wealth of knowledge and experience; and should be your first point of call when in difficulty.

---

### Top tips
### Induction and guidance

If you're going to use flow cytometry, the first thing to do is introduce yourself to the flow technicians in your department or university. Ensure you are fully inducted.

### Controls

You will need to optimise your antibodies through titration, and employ compensation controls, FMO/isotype controls and negative controls in your experiments. Be clear on their differences, what they're there for and how to use them.

**Problem solving**

If your data collection is successful – that is only the beginning. Flow data analysis can be painstaking and error prone. Enlist the help of someone who's experienced to train you up – your whole PhD/paper outcome could depend on this competency alone. In their absence, hit the tutorial videos – hard.

**Heads up**

New antibodies and flow products are released frequently. Keep your head up and aware of developments. Build understanding with sales reps of notable bioscience companies, and take advantage of the copious deals and offers they run to get good value for your reagents.

## Statistics

### Speak to a friendly statistician – early!

The two main statistical questions you are likely to ask are:

1. How big a sample do I need?
2. How should I analyse my data?

You might think that you can safely leave these questions until the project is well underway, perhaps until after you have collected some data. But sometimes the answers to these questions can have a fundamental effect on your research question or objectives. For example, the answer may be that you need more subjects than you can afford or can recruit within 3 years, or that you need to add an extra comparison group to answer the research question. Therefore, it is always a good idea to seek a statistician's advice as early as possible in your PhD journey.

When you've set up your appointment with the statistician, here is the kind of information that will be helpful to bring with you:

- What is the main question and study objective?
- What is your study design (e.g. randomised controlled trial, lab experiment, cohort study, case-control study, cross-sectional survey)?
- What is the exact structure of your study/experiment?
- What is your main outcome measure – and is this numerical, ordinal, or nominal in nature?

If it's an intervention study:

- How many groups do you have (and specifically how many intervention groups, how many control groups)?
- Are your groups independent, paired, or matched?
- How were subjects allocated to groups?

If it's an observational study:
• What are your main predictors?
• What confounding factors will you be adjusting for?

What comparisons do you plan to make, or what are the associations of interest?

## Calculating your sample size

There are a number of online sample size calculators available, or you may have access to a software package that will do this for you. However, it is definitely a good idea to seek advice from an experienced statistician at this point, as it is too important to not get right!

Although your study will almost certainly be aiming to perform many analyses, the sample size calculation will generally relate to the single, most important analysis of your primary outcome. All sample size calculations need to be 'fed' with relevant information. Let's take one of the most common types of analysis as an example – the comparison of the means for two groups. This will require four pieces of information:

• An estimate of the standard deviation of the variable being compared – *this could be obtained from your own previous work, or from similar work in the literature, or by conducting a small preliminary study*
• The smallest size of difference between the means which would be clinically important, or biologically meaningful – *this is not a 'statistical' decision, rather it is a judgement that you or your supervisor should make*
• The significance level of the proposed significance test – *usually 0.05*
• The power of the proposed significance test – *usually 0.8 for preliminary studies, and 0.9 for definitive trials*

A typical sample size statement in your dissertation will include this information; for example – 'A sample size of 133 in each group will be sufficient to detect a difference of 2 units in Serum X, between groups A and B, with 90% power, at a 5% significance level, assuming Serum X has a standard deviation of 5 units.'

Don't forget to factor in an allowance for any drop-outs; so, for example, if you expect 10% of your sample to be lost or drop out before completing the study, then you should increase the initial sample size accordingly (e.g. in the example here, you would start with 148 in each group).

## Analysing your data
### Describing your data

You will probably want to start with some descriptive statistics, to display the key characteristics of your sample. For numerical variables, the mean and standard deviation will provide measures of the centre and spread of your data respectively, or if your data are notably skewed (rather than symmetric), then the median and interquartile range are a suitable alternative. For categorical variables, the number and percentage in each category can be presented. In addition, think about giving a measure of the precision of your sample means or percentages (the larger your sample, the more precise your estimate) – in lab sciences, the standard error is usually given, while clinical sciences favour 95% confidence intervals. Graphs, such as boxplots or bar charts can also be a useful way of presenting descriptive statistics.

### Testing your hypotheses

Your next stage will usually be to test some hypotheses using statistical significance tests. The purpose of such tests is to provide a $p$-value, which tells you the probability of observing a difference as large (or larger) as that found in your sample data, if there is actually no real difference in the underlying population (or in colloquial terms, the probability you could have observed these results 'by chance'). A $p$-value of less than 0.05 is generally taken to be sufficiently small to allow you to conclude that a real difference does indeed exist, and we call this a statistically significant result.

### Choosing a test

Some of the most common statistical significance tests are:
- Independent samples t-test – for comparing the means of two independent groups
- Paired samples t-test – for comparing the means of two paired groups
- Analysis of variance (or ANOVA) – for comparing the means of three or more independent groups
- Chi-squared test and Fisher's exact test – for comparing percentages between (any number of) independent groups
- McNemar's test – for comparing percentages between two paired groups
- Correlation coefficient – for assessing the association between two numerical variables

### Checking your test assumptions

All significance tests have assumptions that must be checked, otherwise they may not be valid. For example, some tests require the data to be normally distributed. You can check this by simply plotting a histogram of your data, or there are specific tests (e.g. the Kolmogorov–Smirnov test) that you can use to check for normality. However, caution is needed when interpreting such tests, particularly with small samples, where the results are often inconclusive.

### Do you need a non-parametric test?

If the assumptions of your chosen test cannot be verified, you might consider a non-parametric test, which makes no assumptions about the distribution of numerical variables. For example, the Mann–Whitney-U test is a non-parametric alternative to the independent samples t-test. Non-parametric tests tend to be less 'powerful' than their parametric equivalents (i.e. less likely to find statistically significant results). So, another approach would be to find a mathematical transformation which will turn your skewed dataset into a normally distributed dataset, allowing you to continue with parametric tests, such as the t-test. For positively skewed data, the log transformation is always worth trying.

### Adding in other variables

All the tests described so far are 'unifactorial', that is, they look for an association between one outcome variable, and one explanatory or predictor variable. If you want to see whether your outcome is related to several predictors at the same time, you will need a 'multifactorial' approach. This can be done via different forms of multiple regression modelling, including:

• Linear regression – for numerical outcomes
• Logistic regression – for binary (yes/no) outcomes
• Cox regression – for 'time-to-event' outcomes, like survival data

   Typically, you would use these methods when conducting an observational study (e.g. cohort or cross-sectional study), where you need to adjust for confounding factors, or for a randomised controlled trial if you have used a stratified randomisation method.

### Doing something different, or more complex?

The most common forms of statistical analysis involve comparing an outcome measure between treatment groups or between risk factors, or looking for associations between variables. But there are a multitude of different study designs that require their own special methods of analysis – for example, studies of diagnostic accuracy; agreement between two methods of measurement; multi-level models; survival analysis; meta-analysis; cluster randomised trials … for which you should knock on the door of that friendly statistician!

### Improving your statistical skills

Your university should offer some postgraduate research training sessions in statistics, which are also a good place to meet some statistics lecturers who might be able to give you further advice. In addition, there may be funding available to attend a formal university short course in statistics, and there are usually preferential rates for students. Try to identify the most relevant course for your particular project – for example, if you are conducting a clinical trial, there are specific courses which relate to the statistical analysis of trials.

   Your university should have statistical software which you can access. Common software packages used by postgraduate students include SPSS,

Stata and GraphPad Prism. The former two packages are mainly used for the clinical sciences, and the latter for lab sciences. There are a multitude of statistics books available for the biomedical and health sciences – see the 'Further reading' list at the end of this section.

---

### Top tips

- *Multiple testing*: Beware the dangers of 'multiple testing', where you test many exploratory hypotheses, or analyse many subgroups – this will result in over-optimistic $p$-values. You should either avoid it, or adjust for it (e.g. by the Bonferroni correction), or at least report how many tests you have performed.

- *Outliers*: If you have outliers in your data, consider analysing your data both with and without the outliers (a sensitivity analysis), and reporting both sets of results.

- *Independent observations*: A basic requirement of statistical tests is that all the observations are independent. If you have repeated measures on any subject (e.g. left and right limbs; or measures repeated over time), this will need to be factored appropriately into your analysis.

---

## References

1. Nicholson, J.K., Lindon, J.C., Holmes E. (1999) 'Metabolomics': understanding the metabolic responses of living systems to pathophysiological stimuli via multivariate statistical analysis of biological NMR spectroscopic data. *Xenobiotica* Nov;29(11):1181–1189.
2. Worley, B, Powers, R. (2013) Multivariate analysis in metabolomics. *Curr Metabolomics* 1(1):92–107.

## Further reading

### Genomics

1. Bunyavanich, S., Schadt, E.E. (2015) 'Systems biology of asthma and allergic diseases: a multiscale approach.' *J Allergy Clin Immunol.* 135(1):31–42.
2. Coughlin, S.S. (2014) 'Toward a road map for global -omics: a primer on -omic technologies' *Am J Epidemiol.* 180(12):1188–1195.
3. Valdes, A.M., Glass, D., Spector, T.D. (2013) 'Omics technologies and the study of human ageing' *Nat Rev Genet.* 14(9):601–607.

### Metabolomics

1. Cockerell, G.L., McKim, J.M., Vonderfecht, S.L. (2002) Strategic importance of research support through pathology. *Toxicol Pathol* 30(1):4–7.

2. Nicholson, J.K., Lindon, J.C., Holmes E. (1999) 'Metabolomics': understanding the metabolic responses of living systems to pathophysiological stimuli via multivariate statistical analysis of biological NMR spectroscopic data. *Xenobiotica* Nov;29(11):1181–1189.
3. Worley, B, Powers, R. (2013) Multivariate analysis in metabolomics. *Curr Metabolomics* 1(1):92–107.

## Flow cytometry

1. Jahan-Tigh, R.R., Ryan, C., Obermoser, G., Schwarzenberger, K. (2012) Flow cytometry, *J Invest Dermatol.* 132(10):e1.
2. Websites from BD Biosciences (www.bdbiosciences.com/), Invitrogen/Molecular probes (https://www.thermofisher.com/) and Biolegend (www.biolegend.com/) are a good source of information about available fluorochromes and their excitation/emission spectral properties.
3. The spectrum viewer from BD Biosciences is particularly good for designing complex antibody panels (www.bdbiosciences.com/eu/s/spectrumviewer).

## Statistics

1. Petrie, A., Sabin, C. (2009) *Medical Statistics at a Glance*, 3rd Edition. Wiley-Blackwell.
2. Peacock, J., Peacock, P. (2011) *Oxford Handbook of Medical Statistics.* Oxford University Press, Oxford.
3. Bland, M. (2015) *An Introduction to Medical Statistics*, 4th Edition, Oxford University Press, Oxford.
4. Another useful source of information is the many reporting guidelines available for different types of study, which have been collated by the Equator network – see www.equator-network.org/.

# Chapter 5 **Take off: Year 1**

*Ashton Barnett-Vanes[1] and Rachel Allen[2]*

[1] MB-PhD Candidate, St George's, University of London and Imperial College London, UK

[2] Reader in Immunology of Infection and Head of Graduate School, St George's, University of London, UK

## Background

Having chosen to embark on a PhD, identified a supervisor and agreed upon a project, you've actually been working on your PhD for several months. However, this is the first 'real' day in the department – so look sharp.

You'll need to set up your desk, meet key people in your group and building, and undergo the relevant inductions and assessments before you get started. Often these include a lab or area safety induction, an occupational health assessment and possibly the undertaking of specific courses. In some universities, a departmental administrator may be able to help arrange these, if not ask your peers as you're unlikely to be the first to do so. Getting these completed is a priority and you should aim to have most of these appointments made before you start. Give your student handbook a thorough read too, this will spell out the institutional timelines and deadlines ahead of you.

Alongside the introductions, it's important to embed within your university or research institute. You might have studied there previously, or already be pushed with clinical commitments to maintain, but making time to become part of the wider student and research community is worthwhile. A PhD is a marathon not a sprint: clubs, societies and social groups are part of that process and will give you much needed respite from intense months of research, reading or writing. Moreover, your research colleagues may one day be your collaborators or reviewers, building those connections now will be helpful down the line.

*How to Complete a PhD in the Medical and Clinical Sciences,*
First Edition. Edited by Ashton Barnett-Vanes and Rachel Allen.
© 2018 John Wiley & Sons Ltd. Published 2018 by John Wiley & Sons Ltd.

Now you've got the badge it's time to get to work. All supervisors and students will have different perspectives on how the first year should flow. In this chapter, we'll cover the essentials: getting to grips with your project, the Literature, Research proposal, first experiments and 'Transfer'. Ready for take off?

## Understanding your team and project

Often new PhD students in medical science can feel under pressure to get started quickly and show some results. This is a natural feeling, you're new and there's always a desire to demonstrate what you can do. But unlike other degrees or projects, a PhD is 3 or 4 *years*. Whether you're coming from a basic science or clinical background, the foundations you lay in the first year will dictate how the rest unfold.

First, you need to know who's on your team. You'll have a primary and secondary supervisor – you may also have a tertiary supervisor. Ask and then figure out what each of their roles will be, and make sure they all agree. The last thing you need is disharmony among them, hence three should usually be the upper limit. You'll likely have a mentor too, and if you don't go and find one – preferably someone senior to talk to in confidence who's not in your group or closely associated with your supervisors.

Next, it's vital to get to grips with your project as soon as possible. Check what procedures or techniques you'll be performing and importantly what documentation (e.g. licences) are in place before you start. A project licence (necessary to start a new project involving research on humans or animals) can take up to 6 months to be processed and approved: start early.

Too often, PhD students in their first year find it difficult to explain what they're doing or why they're even there. This could be because your project outline has largely been dictated to you, or because you haven't yet figured out what you're going to do. Neither situations are a problem so long as you take ownership, fast. For example, key project questions to ask yourself are: what is the project trying to achieve? Why are you doing it this way? Who else has done this or something similar? Other important questions may include: where will you be working? What support is there around me? Are there collaborators? Is there someone to teach me new techniques? How do I order consumables? And so on. Some of these will have been covered at the interview stage (see Chapter 2); however, it is not uncommon for these details to change between your summer interview and winter start date. These questions must be addressed before you can meaningfully start to explore the literature and write a strong research proposal.

## The literature

Getting to know the literature in a medical or clinical science PhD is daunting and laborious. There are tens of thousands of articles and it is one of the fastest proliferating fields. So, the first thing you need is a strategy. Picture or draw a diagram of the key themes in your project and where they intersect. For example, you might have three key themes of: ventilator-induced lung injury, neutrophils and inflammation. Sub-divide these into their composite parts (three or four each). You should now have a set of around 10 key words or concepts associated with your project. When you conduct searches of the literature these key (and eventually sub-key) words will come in handy – see Figure 5.1 for an example.

The literature is composed of several broad groups: journal articles, books and abstracts. These may be online, offline (usually older publications that haven't been digitalised) or both. Your university should have helpful resources for accessing these on and off-site, such as the use of a Virtual Portal Network (VPN). Journal articles will consist of original research articles, reviews, perspectives or editorials. Recent reviews in your area are invaluable, as they'll have sought to encapsulate current understanding. However, these should not be treated as complete. As a result, original research articles are likely to form the core of your PhD literature. These will present research that offers new understanding or perspectives, and you should become familiar with the relevant work (recent and seminal) quickly. Books are helpful, especially for learning new techniques, but there are few for cutting edge research as these often become quickly outdated. Finally, abstracts and conference proceedings can give you glimpses of what other

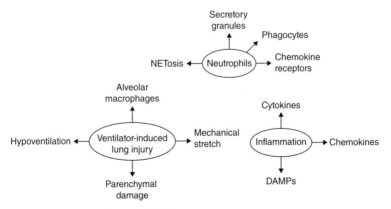

**Figure 5.1** Literature key word mind map

groups are doing, and what results they have found. However, these often lack detail and make interpretation of the data and conclusions challenging; Chapter 8 covers publishing in journals.

Searching the literature can be done manually or via the use of specific software (Table 5.1). PubMed is a common source for medical and clinical science journals, but there are many journals not indexed in PubMed. Software such as GoogleScholar can facilitate deeper searching within the text of an article, and signpost articles that have since cited it. Utilise your search terms, alone or in combination to find the right information and always follow the references in a paper. There are functions available to get newly published papers that match your key words automatically emailed to you. It's worthwhile registering for the weekly or monthly Table of Contents (ToC) from journals very relevant to your project or using RSS feeds.

**Table 5.1** Common literature search software

| Name | Website | Comment |
|------|---------|---------|
| OvidSP | http://ovidsp.ovid.com/ | ✓ Powerful search facility that enables you to search a range of key words and terms; particularly good for systematic reviews.<br>– Often requires institutional access. |
| PubMed | www.ncbi.nlm.nih.gov/pubmed | ✓ Free to use, this website indexes a range of scientific and clinical journals from the world's most reputable journals; particularly good at following an author's published work.<br>– Many articles and journals are not indexed in PubMed. |
| Google Scholar | https://scholar.google.co.uk/ | ✓ Free to use, this works as a tailored search engine to bring key search terms and publications; very helpful to track papers that have cited an article of interest.<br>– Can produce overwhelmingly large numbers of search results if using undescriptive search terms. |
| Search engines | https://www.google.co.uk/ https://uk.search.yahoo.com/ https://www.bing.com/ | ✓ Free to use, often work by tracking the search terms in the html text of the journal articles; very good for finding papers whose title you can only remember half of; can occasionally pull specific sections of pertinent text out of an article in the search results.<br>– Not so helpful if searching old publications which are digitally archived as PDFs. |
| Hybrid eg Papers | www.papersapp.com/ | ✓ Enable the combined search of articles from a range of search facilities.<br>– May require personal or institutional licences/subscription. |

However you choose to search, make sure you can store, organise and retrieve articles efficiently. Save each file as a PDF with the first author surname, title, year of publication and abbreviated journal title. Organise your files, be it by subject area or type of research. Finally, rather than printing off reams of paper, investing in a tablet or smartphone with a cloud-based system enables easy retrieval when at meetings or working. There are apps and software that can help you achieve this (Table 5.2).

## The research proposal

Now you've defined your project and become familiar with the pertinent literature, you'll soon be expected to generate a research proposal or plan (usually within the first 2–3 months). This may be required of you by your university department, funders or supervisor, and represents an opportunity to consolidate your ideas onto a page.

Typically, you'll require an Introduction, Project Aims, Plan of Investigation, timeline and Reference list. The length may vary but 4–8 pages with or without preliminary data (if you have any) would be a reasonable ballpark. The purpose of the research proposal is to ensure what you're thinking is sensible, appropriate and achievable with your resources and time limits. Often these are 'reviewed' by internal examiners who make comments. Supervisors will be keen to ensure the research proposal is strong, and you should leverage this to your advantage by asking all the questions we covered earlier should you still not be clear on any aspect of the task ahead.

Drafting your research proposal serves as a first opportunity to test run your writing, citing and organising skills. You'll need to cite articles in your

**Table 5.2** Literature storage apps and reference managing software

| Name | Website | Comment |
|---|---|---|
| Papers App | www.papersapp.com/ | • Includes literature search, storage and citation functions. |
| EndNote | http://endnote.com/ | • Includes literature search, storage and citation functions. |
| Dropbox | https://www.dropbox.com/ | • Permits storage and syncing of literature across devices. |
| RefWorks | https://www.refworks.com/ | • Includes literature storage and citation functions. |
| Reference Manager | http://refman.com | • Includes literature search, storage and citation functions with a focus on multi-user capabilities. |
| Mendeley | https://www.mendeley.com/ | • Includes literature storage, citation and network functions. |

proposal – it is strongly advised at this stage to pick and stick to a citation/reference manager (Table 5.2). These systems work by organising your references online or offline, allowing you to cite them easily in the text as a placeholder which you can convert to a bibliography as required. Thus, should you need to rearrange paragraphs and text (not uncommon), your citations flexibly follow and you can instantly generate an updated bibliography. Your university may have institutional access or offers on specific programmes for this purpose. Scientific writing comes naturally to some more than others and this is a good time to access any additional assistance should you be struggling. Support courses are commonly run for students whose first language is not English, or for native speakers who encounter difficulty; your university library should be the first point of call. Don't be shy, speak up, you're much better off tackling these sorts of issues now rather than later: your thesis won't write itself.

The specific contents of the proposal will vary between institutions. However, all usually contain a background to the project (why is it important, why is it relevant), hypothesis and central research questions, clearly linked aims and expected milestones. You may be required to defend or present the research proposal to your internal examiners, group or department (see Chapter 8 for 'How to Present'). This can be daunting but remember most PhD theses end up looking very different from the first plan, that's what research is about. People are therefore not looking to be wowed by your proposal and ambitious aims, but for a thorough understanding of the subject area and gaps in the literature, together with some reasoning as to how you intend to address them. Who knows, you might even find a few people wanting to collaborate by the end.

## Starting experiments

Experiments will be your *raison d'être* in a medical and clinical science PhD. These can take myriad of forms, from cell culturing to gait analysis of elite athletes. Yet, there is a common path to follow and it starts with preparation.

As a first year, you may be working alongside others when you start, or at least be shown what to do (if you haven't been, then ask for it). There are three components to getting an experiment to work: knowledge of the protocol and materials, competency in conducting the required techniques, and the gift of experience. You can master the first two quickly, but knowing the intricacies of your work takes time - so watch seniors closely.

At a minimum, you will need to organise and prepare subjects (cells, plants, animals, humans) for your study. Have purchased, reconstituted and optimised all the necessary materials (buffers, electrodes, medias, surgical tools, the list can be endless so make a checklist). Much of this information will be detailed in company and lab protocols which you should access and become familiar with in advance. You may also need to book equipment for processing your samples, or for the analysis (e.g. microscopes, flow cytometers, mass spectrometers). Lastly, you will need to liaise and organise with other people and their time schedules, so plan experiments weeks if not months in advance wherever possible. Too often PhD students dampen their expectations of the first year-'The first year doesn't count' is commonly muttered sympathetically by peers, but this need not be the case. Use the first experiments to learn the best practice, solid knowledge and understanding now will make all the difference in a year's time. Most experiments don't 'work' for one of two reasons: you didn't do it right, or it's not supposed to. You should aim to have always done it right.

Productivity is also very important, the quicker you get things done accurately, the more you can achieve in this and subsequent years. Make experiment days easier by labelling all your materials in advance. Your PhD is much like a 9–5 job, only you have a lot more say over the schedule. Keep active, if you're in the lab for half the day spend the other half reading or in discussion. Work around group and departmental meetings. If you feel you've got nothing to do, something is wrong. Inevitably you'll encounter problems; patients might not show up; you might accidentally throw your cells away or realise you never had any to begin with. These are opportunities to learn from what went wrong, and quickly bounce back. Cautious pessimism and endless optimism are key ingredients for experimental success.

## Data management and record keeping

Three years is over 1000 days of research. Most of these will involve you doing something, be it a full-blown experiment or a casual chat with co-workers. As the tasks begin to accumulate, accurate documentation of what you've done, where and how is vital. Many PhD students have a lab book for this purpose. Everybody uses it differently, but you should aim to make an entry for each substantive task you do. These can be concise, such as 'Changed Media of Cells', so long as you previously defined what 'Media' and what 'Cells' for this particular experiment. At the minimum, you should note the date and time together with a description of the task; keep track of all your product orders and reagents – this can be particularly helpful in triangulating an experimental problem down the line.

When making entries for experiments, it's valuable to include details on the background to your thinking at the time, why and how you did them (e.g. which protocol used), what the results showed and your next steps. This will aid your memory when writing up your thesis. Many students like to print and stick out a summary of their experimental results, however, if yours is 8 hours' worth of EEG recordings, this may be inappropriate. Photocopy your lab book periodically as a back-up. You should also make notes of meetings with supervisors and colleagues. Note down the pertinent areas, and always clarify the action points going forwards. Once you get back to your desk, summarise this as an email and send it to all meeting participants interested: you now have a written and digital document of the meeting.

As you progress through your first year you'll accumulate all kinds of data, which depending on the type could be very large. For example, an excel spreadsheet of ELISA or PCR values will differ enormously in size from a mass spectrometry analysis. So, ensure you've got the data storage facilities you need. These may include data hard drives on your computer, external hard drives, secure university network drives or cloud-based storage. You should ensure your data is backed up (e.g. home and work computers), well organised and secure. This is your responsibility, supervisors and colleagues often expect this as a given and your university or funding body may have specific requirements for data storage, particularly if it involves patient data. Furthermore, journals can ask to see all kinds of data when considering an article – you don't want to drop the ball at that stage.

## The 'transfer'

Depending on your institution the name of this process may vary. While traditionally known as a 'transfer' or upgrade, some now refer to it as an early or first year review/assessment. Irrespective of the name, this process typically happens 9–12 months after starting your PhD. It seeks to assess whether what you've done, and critically what you *intend* to do, will be sufficient to be considered for the award of a PhD. Usually this will require a substantive report including data and a presentation. The report will likely be in the typical research article format with a few additions*: Introduction, Aims/Hypothesis*, Methods, Results, Discussion, Conclusions and Future Work*. Length will vary but anything up to 30–40 pages in total would be reasonable. Given the time this will require to write, it's worthwhile laying the foundations of your final thesis in this process. And while most students won't have many concrete results at this stage, the Introduction and methods could form your thesis outline, given by now you should have got to grips with the existing literature relevant to your project. Making a ToC is required and can be expedited significantly by utilising the styles function in Microsoft Word or the equivalent in another word processing package. This function enables you to assign specific headings, subheadings and text formats quickly and has a built-in ToC generating function (see Chapter 9 for further formatting tips). Again, like a citation manager, this will trim hours off your writing time and offers you the flexibility to reorder and change whole sections as needed. Once complete, keep adding to this over the following year, as you'll be in a much stronger position to start writing your thesis. You could also look towards submitting the literature review aspect of your transfer as a journal review. Discuss this with your supervisor in advance.

In the report and transfer presentation/viva, your examiners are looking for evidence that you know what you're trying to do, and have the necessary time and resources available to do it. Some data will be required, if it's negative that's not necessarily a problem so long as you have reasons as to why and a plan going forwards. If you haven't got any results, don't know the literature and have no plan, you are likely to be called for a review. This may entail a probation period or a request to 'downgrade' to an MPhil or the equivalent. While this happens in only a minority of cases, it is possible, so take the transfer seriously. We cover the process of presenting during your PhD in Chapter 8. But for your research proposal at this stage, people are looking for understanding of the problem and sound methods to try and address it. You are not expected to have *Nature* quality data by now (well done if you do).

## Conclusion

The first year of your PhD should be one of the most enjoyable. It's the time where you are new, and the demands and expectations placed on you will be modest compared to later years. Striking a balance and implementing good practice early with respect to reading, writing and data management will leave you in a good position. While the majority of students get through their first year relatively unscathed, some will find it particularly challenging.

## Common pitfalls

We hereby outline a few common pitfalls associated with the first year; however, dealing with problems associated with your PhD is covered extensively later in Chapter 6.

1. *'None of my experiments are working I have no data.'*
   This is a common situation first (and at times second and third!) year PhD students encounter. As discussed, there are usually only a few reasons why an experiment doesn't 'work'. Ensure you're documenting everything you do so should things change you can triangulate what might have helped.

If you're concerned about your competency, seek help from post-docs or students with the right skills. If you're worried the aim is not right, talk to your supervisor or mentor. But don't keep doing the same thing for 6 months, you don't have the time to waste.

2. *'I don't want to be here – I'm already counting down the days.'*
There are occasions where PhD students realise they don't want to be there. Problem is, unlike a typical degree where one can 'drop out' relatively easily, a PhD is a bit like a job. You effectively have a contract with your department and/or funders, including substantial resource allocation. If the thought is fleeting, stick at it as you wouldn't have done all the work to get here if you weren't committed. If, however, you cannot escape the feeling, weigh up the time and money and consider whether you can downgrade. Be warned though, this may be at the discretion of others.

3. *'I want a* Nature *publication before the end of my first year and haven't slept in a month.'*
It is important to start off strong in a PhD, but as mentioned it is a marathon not a sprint. Working too intensely in your first year may leave you burnt out for subsequent years. High ambitions are good but brace yourself - science is unpredictable. You need to be prepared for long-term and infrequent 'rewards' as much as out of the blue successes. If you don't manage to get a *Nature* publication by Year 2, life will go on…

4. *'I'd rather be gathering data than keeping a lab book or writing progress or transfer reports that don't matter.'*
It's quite normal to want to get into the lab or clinic and get data, especially if your study subjects are rare. However, instituting good practices in all the domains of your PhD will ensure you can succeed without hindrance. You

---

### Top tips

1. Understanding your project – make your introduction appointments in advance where possible to save time.
2. The Literature – utilise search software and get ToCs delivered to your email to keep abreast even when you're not actively searching.
3. Starting experiments – learn new techniques quickly by becoming familiar with the relevant protocols in advance.
4. Record keeping – institute good practices with your lab book early to leave less to do at the writing up stage.
5. Transfer – use your literature review in your transfer as the basis for a review article to be submitted for publication on your research area.

could be doing exceptional work or already have found something novel, but if you don't write a good report or complete your checkpoints on time you will run into problems. Furthermore, these can be helpful junctions for reflecting on your progress and receiving feedback from peers and supervisors. Remember, the administrators of your department will have their own results to report about your progress: tick those boxes already!

5. *'It'll sort itself out – everybody gets their PhD, right?'*
   One thing that you cannot afford to do in your PhD is back off and expect things to just happen. Just as you wouldn't expect someone else to push your trolley in a supermarket, don't expect anyone to push your project along for you. It requires maintained effort, be constructive when you're encountering difficulty. Project apathy will not get you far.

# Chapter 6 **Dealing with problems**

*Rachel Allen[1] and David Salman[2]*
[1] Reader in Immunology of Infection and Head of Graduate School, St George's, University of London, UK
[2] Wellcome Trust Clinical Research Training Fellow, Imperial College London, UK

## Background

As a degree based upon an independent and novel research project, a PhD will be a very different experience for each student. It's not surprising then, that many describe their PhD as being a lonely and difficult experience at times. A simple internet search using the terms 'PhD' and 'mental illness' identifies a wide range of articles and blogs concerning the problems students face, revealing how common it is for PhD students to struggle with anxiety and depression, perhaps to a greater extent than most other student groups. Indeed, a survey of PhD students at one UK university revealed that about 40% of them believed studying for a doctorate had worsened their physical and mental health[1]. This chapter will discuss some of the common problems that can arise, and to which even the most resilient PhD student is not immune: your study design might turn out to be inappropriate, experiments fail for unknown reasons or your relationship with your supervisor might deteriorate. Many students try to tough it out; others may change their project or supervisors entirely; some may even drop out.

A key skill for maintaining the resilience you'll need to survive a PhD is some personal insight into your own tendencies – are you a perfectionist or a procrastinator? Do you need a lot of structure in order to feel secure? Are you competitive or prone to self-criticism? Such understanding can help you to identify when your tendencies might affect your PhD progress, and how to develop the ability to control them.

*How to Complete a PhD in the Medical and Clinical Sciences,*
First Edition. Edited by Ashton Barnett-Vanes and Rachel Allen.
© 2018 John Wiley & Sons Ltd. Published 2018 by John Wiley & Sons Ltd.

## General problems

### Work-life balance

By the time you begin your PhD, you'll have at least one other degree under your belt. You may be a scientist hopping from a BSc or MSc; however, if you're a clinician, you may have spent a while away from full-time academic study. Either way, you'll be older than undergraduate students and likely to have different life priorities or concerns regarding your future career. While you may have already considered the impact of a PhD on your life priorities, you'll want to keep these under review as you progress through the years of PhD study.

Typically, a PhD is a full-time working experience, but it should not be all-consuming or at the expense of your life or health. Neglecting these impacts may buy you time in the short-term, but will most likely adversely affect the quality of your life, and work, in the long-term. A simple time audit (Table 6.1), assessing how much you spend on various activities including socialising, family life, exercise and so on, as well as your work, can help you decide where your time needs to be prioritised to balance competing demands. Sometimes, of course, you'll have to focus on one area at the expense of another (for many people this comes at the final stages of their PhD), but a prolonged imbalance is not sustainable and risks you burning out. Make sure that you give yourself the breaks that you need to maintain your physical and mental health. Engaging in sports and exercise will not only increase your social network during what can be quite an isolating experience, it will keep you fit and add some crucial structure to your day (see next) – some of your best ideas may appear during a swim or run!

This table shows a simple time audit, where you can enter the hours spent each day on a particular activity. Following this over a week or so should

**Table 6.1** How to do a time audit

| Activity | Time per day/week (hours) |
| --- | --- |
| Sleeping | |
| Commuting | |
| Work/Study | |
| Socialising at work | |
| (coffee breaks, lunch, office conversations) | |
| Socialising outside work | |
| Home and family commitments | |
| Eating | |
| Relaxation and 'time out' | |
| Exercise/fitness | |

reveal the areas which need attention and help you allocate your time. As your PhD progresses, you may find it helpful to break the work/study category down into different subsections (e.g. experiments, reading, writing) to ensure that you're giving appropriate time to each.

Although studying for a PhD is an exercise in dealing with problems, life does not go on hold when you are working towards one, and there are situations you should not be expected to overcome alone.

### Personal difficulties

If you unfortunately suffer a setback that may interfere with your work, such as prolonged ill-health or bereavement, it is important to inform your university, supervisors and possibly funding body at the earliest opportunity. This will allow such circumstances to be taken into account when planning your research, progression towards obtaining your degree, and funding. It may be possible to change from full-time PhD programme milestones to part-time ones, to allow for some breathing space; alternatively, you can interrupt your studies for an agreed period to allow you to recover. If you do interrupt your studies, make sure that you discuss what will happen to your stipend during this period. Several universities offer support in the form of a postgraduate tutor and mentorship programme; who can provide a safe arena in which to discuss issues in confidence with impartiality and with a view to building practical solutions.

### Financial difficulties

It is in your university's interest that you can concentrate and succeed in your work. Therefore, although it is sensible to plan for the period of reduced income that a PhD often entails through a simple audit, see Table 6.2, should you find yourself in financial difficulty, you can approach this in the same way as described above, talking in the first instance with your supervisor. Indeed, many universities offer a 'financial advice' service, which is there to help you. There may also be the opportunity to access hardship funds, such as one-off student support funds that may not need to be repaid. Engaging in some proactive financial planning prior to starting your PhD can help identify potential problems in advance, and may pay dividends down the line.

Calculate your monthly stipend and compare this against the totals from Table 6.1. Although you can take into consideration any savings you have which can support you during your PhD – aim to live within your monthly income. Bear in mind that income from teaching activities and so on can fluctuate from month to month. Try to save some money if you can – many students end up supporting themselves through a month or two of 'writing up' before moving on to their next job.

**Table 6.2** A PhD student's financial audit

| Income | Amount (per month) |
| --- | --- |
| Monthly stipend/grant | |
| Other income (e.g. teaching) | |
| **Outgoings** | |
| Rent | |
| Bills | |
| Groceries | |
| Holidays | |
| Socialising | |
| Savings | |
| Debt repayments | |
| **Net surplus/deficit** | |

## Loneliness

At some point, someone will have told you to expect to become the leading expert in your immediate project area by the end of your PhD. But nobody will tell you about the individual trials and tribulations you'll face on your way to this said exalted position! Fellow PhD students and post-docs will have some understanding though. In the UK, there is a move towards establishing cohorts of PhD students who train together to provide the necessary peer support and collaborative networks. When building or maintaining your peer network, it's also worth bearing in mind where you might all end up in the future – reviewing grants or editing journals for example. Building strong connections might benefit you long after your PhD. Loneliness may be further compounded by home sickness if you've moved to a new environment and away from home support networks. It is important to try and build social networks in your university and beyond. Social events can help you forget (hopefully briefly) about things, put them in context, and provide you with some much needed respite. If you feel that your problems need additional help, many institutions provide access to free counselling services. Finally, if you notice that these feelings are affecting your appetite or sleep, then speak to a General Medical Practitioner.

## Academic problems

### Assessing your progress against peers

If you've succeeded in obtaining a PhD scholarship and registering for the degree, you're likely to be a high achiever who has performed well in previous academic exams. Life as a PhD student is a very different academic environment, where you'll no longer be examined at regular intervals. Not many people enjoy sitting exam after exam alongside their peers, but these can provide a source of comfort or a wake-up call that is absent from a PhD. It's important to be aware of your tendencies – will you struggle without the reassurance from regular assessment that you're doing OK or without a benchmark for comparison with your peers?

That said, it's advisable to avoid the temptation to compare yourself with fellow students to assess how well you are doing. Everyone has a different project with its own unique cycle of progress and delays. Further, the level of success a project may attain often depends on how established the lab or group is in the field; high impact publications require more than a single capable PhD student, and therefore should not be seen as a barometer of your 'ability' or progress. Moreover, avoid the trap of falling into excessive competition with yourself, be it five first author publications or a 'perfect' PhD thesis; while it's important to set yourself challenges, be realistic and recognise science is a fluid field that cannot be controlled. Supervisors and examiners will expect you to learn and develop over the course of your degree. If you lean towards perfectionism, a PhD will help you negotiate with what is 'good enough'. All scientific work will have shortcomings, indeed discussing these will form an essential part of your thesis and viva.

## Lack of structure

Three years can seem a very long time at the outset of a PhD. Scientific discovery is difficult to timetable, and as time progresses, you may find yourself deviating further from your original project plans. If you're aware that you need reassurance from structure, or if the scale of a 3-year research project seems overwhelming, break things down into short-term work plans with achievable goals. You can review these with your supervisors at regular intervals to put them in context and plan out the next phase. Another way of providing structure is to establish weekly work routines. So, alongside your research, you assign blocks of time towards writing or data assessment on particular days of the week, along with regular journal clubs, lab meetings and so on. For example, you may want to dedicate Fridays to lab book maintenance (or rehabilitation) and literature reading. Many postgraduate schools offer courses on time management – these are helpful in reinforcing proactive as opposed to reactive behaviours.

## Procrastination

Structuring your time will also help you combat procrastination, a common trap of PhD study. Those who have previously relied on exams and deadlines to scare them into action can struggle to motivate themselves consistently during their PhD. Obviously, cramming a PhD into the final 3 months of a 36-month course is impossible. And so a cycle of procrastination can ensue – where your work is half-paced with a dull anxiety lingering in the back of your mind. Moments of stress, such as when your supervisor demands to see some actual results or as a presentation approaches, can force you to set unrealistic 'catch up' targets. Failure to hit these can lead to a sense of guilt or failure.

At its worst, this cycle can become debilitating, leading PhD students to avoid supervisors and colleagues as well as their work amid spiralling anxiety and depression[2]. If you find yourself drifting towards this state, seek assistance as soon as possible. Further, steer away from fellow procrastinators and their 3-hour coffee breaks, in case this amplifies your own behaviour. Instead, use colleagues (and a degree of peer pressure) as a tool to motivate yourself. It can help to set up informal groups who work together, for example, going to a coffee shop together for an hour of dedicated writing or data analysis, with a suitable reward at the end (cake). Ultimately, a key driver of procrastination is an avoidance of the scale of the research task that lies in wait. It is daunting, particularly given how unclear the road ahead often appears. However, the sooner this is confronted, the quicker you'll be able to feel a sense of control and agency over your PhD.

### Fear of criticism

This is another common issue for PhD students, whether they fall into the categories of high achievers, perfectionists or the overly self-critical. Nobody enjoys being criticised, but listening and responding constructively to criticism is something that every PhD student will have to come to terms with in order to survive their viva. It's also an essential skill for anyone who wants to undertake a research career, and for (married) life generally. After all, publications and grant applications are assessed by peer review, albeit in a less immediately stressful manner than a viva. Delivering research seminars and conference presentations will accustom you to responding to outside opinions of your work. If this seems daunting, start with smaller presentations to your research group or to other students. Bear in mind that you're developing your skills through this process – the more you do it, the more you'll become acclimatised to criticism and the better you'll get at responding to it. Finally, remind yourself that criticism of your work is not criticism of you as a person. By the time you reach your viva, you'll have invested years of your life into the work presented in your thesis and this emotional connection can make it particularly hard to deal with criticism, however well-intended or appropriate. With time and experience, the distinction between your personal and professional identities will become clearer.

### Building resilience

So, what can you do to help yourself survive the polytrauma of a PhD? When you feel under stress, and especially during the final months, ensure that you're eating well, getting some exercise and taking enough time out each day to enable yourself to think and work effectively. These points may sound obvious but it's easy to become so wrapped up in your work that they fall by the wayside – so check them as a priority whenever things start to become a struggle. Be honest with yourself about any confidence and self-esteem issues, and if necessary, ask a trusted friend whether you are being over-critical or overgenerous about your work. Check whether you are jumping to conclusions or personalising issues unnecessarily. A supportive supervisor or mentor should also be able to provide you with the necessary feedback – what you are doing well and what needs more attention.

Adaptability is an important skill for every PhD student. Try as much as you can to keep a sense of humour through the bad times as well as the good. A positive but realistic outlook will make you a better colleague, who finds it easier to access support. You will encounter pressure during your PhD; this can be motivating and may help you through a phase of intense work. When you pass beyond pressure into severe stress, losing concentration and falling into a cycle of negative thoughts, take some time out to think through the issues; get some self-insight; and if necessary, seek advice and support from your peers – whatever works best for you. Your university will provide various support systems: counselling services, mentors and graduate school staff. They're there for a reason, so take advantage of them. Importantly, they'll have dealt with many PhD students in difficult situations and can provide valuable support and reassurance. You can also check to see whether your university has peer support networks such as StudentMinds[3] or set up one of your own. Remember, you do not need to suffer in silence.

## Common PhD problems

### Project title

If you've applied for an advertised studentship, a title for your project will have been in place long before you start. When you embark on your project, the title can be a useful guide of the 'big picture' of what you are aiming to achieve (and to explain to confused relatives what it is that you're doing with 3 years of your life). It can also keep you on track for producing the coherent story that your thesis examiners will expect when they come to read your thesis. That said, the title of your project should not be viewed as a straitjacket but rather as a loose-fitting shirt: it can shift and evolve to fit the direction of your research. If your project changes beyond what was initially expected, then so can the title of your study. If nothing else, you may want to fine-tune it to provide the most appropriate title for your thesis. Alternatively, you may find that your project as you originally envisioned or agreed, is being intentionally transformed in direction or scope, against your will. This can occur, often at the direction of supervisors who feel there's reason to change course – usually in cases where funding is less stringent on specific project aims. There's likely to be a motive and justification for this (perhaps a new publication or finding?), which you should enquire about as early as possible. If you're adamant that you don't want this change in direction to occur, discuss your concerns and justification with your supervisor, and if necessary, director of postgraduate studies. Importantly, one caveat here – regardless of the scenario – concerns ethics; if you have applied for ethical approval, you must undertake the study as originally outlined, or seek further approval if you need to make any changes.

### Project direction

What if, despite your best efforts, a PhD project goes nowhere? This can be a simple matter of bad luck; hypotheses can be wrong or well thought-out experimental approaches may simply not work. A PhD can contain negative data and failed experiments, as long as you are aware of and able to discuss any potential shortcomings of your approach and describe how you tried to address the problems. Some supervisors mitigate for potential failure by running two closely related projects alongside one another, usually one straightforward project which should generate data and another higher-stakes project. This helps maintain some progress when one of them hits delays. Part of a project's success depends on the experience and track record of the group or lab in your field. If you are entering a project where lab protocols are robustly established and published – for example, rigorous flow cytometry in animal models of disease, you will generate data quickly, and rapidly discern what is working and what isn't. If your project is about developing or optimising new models or techniques, be prepared for negative data, and consider how you can document and include them in your thesis. If you find that your project really is doomed, then speak to your supervisor and graduate school staff, who can assist you in devising a suitable alternative if necessary.

### Supervisors

In an ideal world, you'll have an excellent relationship with your supervisor from the start to the finish of your PhD, where they tailor their support as you develop into an independent researcher. In reality, you may at some point encounter challenges: personality clashes, differing expectations, disagreements over the direction or ownership of the project, poor feedback or a lack of support from your supervisor.

Technically, your supervisor is neither a friend nor a mentor because they have a personal vested interest in your 'success'. PhD supervision is a standard job requirement for academics, with their performance assessed during annual reviews and during applications for promotion. They also benefit from authorship on any papers that arise from your degree. This should therefore be considered a mutual relationship, it is your hard work that will contribute to their success, as well as your own. Aim for both sensitivity and perspective between yourself and your supervisor; what seems like a major issue to one party can appear as a minor hitch to the other – with time and understanding this becomes easier. Prepare for each supervisory meeting – arrive with a list of topics that you wish to discuss and specify where you need feedback from them. Keeping a record of meetings is always important and in difficult times can help you confirm mutual understanding of plans and outcomes.

If you hit a rocky patch with your lead supervisor, try first to negotiate with them in a professional manner without personalising any issues. Phonating this can be challenging but it is *your* PhD, be confident while respectful and always aim to keep communication ongoing. If one-on-one meetings are not helping, inviting other members of your supervisory team along as mediators can help by changing the dynamic. You should always have at least two supervisors, see Box 6.1. When these approaches don't improve the situation, it's time to involve other members of staff such as the academics in your department with responsibility for PhD students or graduate school staff. Universities are also assessed on their performance in PhD student completions and are required to provide you with appropriate supervision and support. In the event of a complete breakdown of the student/supervisor relationship it is possible to request a change of supervisor, although such changes, even when handled quickly and smoothly, are likely to result in delays to your completion.

---

**Box 6.1** UK guidance on PhD supervision

- According to latest Quality Assurance Agency (QAA) guidance (4), all PhD students should have at least two supervisors on their project.
- This is to guard against breakdowns in communication with one supervisor, or unexpected events that prevent them from continuing supervision.
- When agreeing supervisors and co-supervisors, be sure to have at least one secondary supervisor. If you are not given the option, raise it with your director of postgraduate studies.

## Colleagues

While we all hope to work amicably with colleagues – in reality, there can always be tension. This is quite natural, given the high-pressure environment collaborative science often creates. However, your aim must be to manage these tensions so as to ensure they do not boil over into clashes. How you do this is largely dependent on the situation and your character. As with supervisors, don't personalise issues unnecessarily and where possible seek perspective from others before you escalate an issue. For example, if someone is using your pipette tips and not replacing them, as frustrating as this may be – it's probably not necessary to involve your head of department. However, if a colleague is repeatedly late for an experiment, or disparaging to your or others – this is worth addressing. Inaction will be perceived as acquiescence.

Challenges may especially arise during interdisciplinary research. This form of research is increasingly becoming the norm in medical and clinical science. However, PhD students or post-docs from other fields (e.g. maths or engineering) may have very different approaches and training, which don't always align with your own. Here, your priority is to proactively troubleshoot and ensure everyone is on the same page. For example, if you don't explain (repeatedly) to an engineer what 'sterile' means, don't be shocked when they walk in the CAT 3 room with steel cap boots and a dirty hardhat. Similarly, what may seem to you like just a few standard deviations, could in fact induce atrial fibrillation in a maths student. Social events, team dinners and the like can help you build common understanding, which can be particularly helpful when it comes to addressing problems.

## Conclusions

There are few other jobs (this is a job after all) that provide the mixture of intellectual liberty and flexibility with the opportunity to be at the forefront of human knowledge. These advantages, however, come at a cost. Finances and personal relationships can suffer, and the seeming lack of structure can lead to uncertainty, procrastination and isolation. Many of the approaches described previously may seem obvious to the unstressed eye. But PhD projects can have a blinkering effect. When your mind is absorbed in research, problems can grow insidiously and present late. Use this chapter and the tool in Box 6.2 as a way to help counter these problems. Finally, though PhD study can feel lonely, the chances are that many others have encountered what you are going through. Your authors certainly have! There exists a wealth of resources to ensure PhD students no longer suffer in silence. We wish you the very best for your PhD.

**Box 6.2** Five steps to deal with any PhD problem

1. *Anticipate*: Identify which problems you're vulnerable to (e.g. lack of structure)
2. *Plan*: Be proactive in avoiding them and recognise your response if they occur
3. *Acknowledge*: Accept when a problem has occurred
4. *Raise it*: Flag your concerns quickly to the appropriate person
5. *Be Systematic*: Try and tackle an issue in a systematic manner, drawing on the breadth of resources available to you in the process

## References

1. Times Higher Educational Supplement. Forty per cent of PhDs at Exeter suffer ill health, study reveals. Available online at: https://www.timeshighereducation.com/news/forty-per-cent-of-phds-at-exeter-suffer-ill-health-study-reveals/2019540.article (accessed 8 December, 2012).
2. Wait But Why. Why procrastinators procrastinate, by Tim Urban. Available online at: http://waitbutwhy.com/2013/10/why-procrastinators-procrastinate.html (accessed 8 December, 2012).
3. Student Minds, The UK's student mental health charity, website: www.studentminds.org.uk/ (accessed 8 December, 2012).

## Further reading

1. QAA, UK Quality Code for Higher Education - Chapter B11: Research degrees. Available online at www.qaa.ac.uk/en/Publications/Pages/Quality-Code-Chapter-B11.aspx#.Vu7r-4Q_UU0 (accessed 8 December, 2012).

# Chapter 7 **Breaking ground: Year 2**

*Ashton Barnett-Vanes[1] and Rebecca Ingram[2]*

[1] MB-PhD Candidate, St George's, University of London and Imperial College London, UK

[2] Lecturer, Queen's University Belfast, UK

## Background

If you are reading this chapter, then you have made it through your PhD transfer/upgrade and – for better or for worse – still want to carry on. The purpose of the first year was to get to grips with your project and develop the skills needed for a lab or clinical research setting; the second year serves somewhat as a transformational period for most PhD students, you're the tadpole that has grown legs, but you're not yet a frog…

PhD students at this stage can feel inadequate in comparison to some of their peers, especially compared to those in their third year, many of whom are benefiting from the transformation you're soon to embark upon. You may have only just got to grips with the techniques used in your project and, despite having done a lot of experiments, few might have actually worked. But fear not, this is a normal and common experience for most PhD students. Indeed, frequently a PhD thesis is predominantly filled with results from the second and/or third year, so it's time to get your head down and really focus.

## Taking ownership of your project

As you launch into the second year, you must become fully immersed in your project. While your supervisor(s) and peers can offer support, ultimately the success of these studies is your responsibility. At the end of your PhD, it will be you who has to justify the research undertaken to your viva examiners. It's likely that your project stems from a grant proposal written by

*How to Complete a PhD in the Medical and Clinical Sciences,*
First Edition. Edited by Ashton Barnett-Vanes and Rachel Allen.
© 2018 John Wiley & Sons Ltd. Published 2018 by John Wiley & Sons Ltd.

your supervisor and/or builds upon previous work in the laboratory. While you may not have had a role in designing this proposal, it's now yours. First years of a PhD can often be or feel overly directed by supervisors. However, as the second year progresses – it's time for you to take over the helm.

A key driver of this transition is your reading and background understanding. While your supervisor will maintain a good grasp of the field and literature, their time commitments and competing projects will restrict the time they can invest in staying abreast of your project area. On the other hand, you should be approaching an enviable level of knowledge around your subject and can draw upon relevant and seemingly unrelated findings to spark new directions for your work. Though your supervisor may still suggest experiments for you to do, you should increasingly be planning the next step. This may seem daunting, so start with small steps. If you include an extra group in your next experiment, will you be able to ask an extra question? If you include an extra marker in the analysis will it tell you something further about the mechanism that you are investigating? And if required, can you draw on the literature to justify your decision?

Time management and prioritising skills will be crucial to making the most of your second year. You might have a funder report due, a conference coming up and your supervisor clamouring to see the latest data set. But can you really, successfully, do all those experiments simultaneously in the one day? Remember, the turtle wins the race: better to do two experiments correctly than ruin four. It's likely that you will be expected to go on some university run training days as part of your PhD – project or time management courses can be useful. Be smart and organise yourself digitally using synced calendars across your desktop, laptop and smartphone. There are particular smartphone apps for this purpose; but if sticky notes are your thing - go to town, so long as you're clear on your priorities for each day and the time you've got allocated to address them. But while taking ownership is crucial, it won't be of much use if you're not ready to start directing where your project is going.

## Shaping the research direction

As you progress through your second year, it's important you begin to build a clear outline of where your project is heading and the sort of data you'll need to form your thesis. It's worth mentioning that while we all enjoy making data, it should be indulged in some moderation; generating huge amounts of unnecessary or inconsequential data is no better than generating nothing at all. Each of your experiments must meet the simple criteria: is this part of, or working towards, something that I could include in my thesis?

Start first by taking some time to sketch out how your thesis might look. Though it varies from institution to institution, all will require: an Introduction, experimental results chapters and a final discussion. Your results are a thesis' centre of gravity, around which other chapters will take shape. So, start with these. Do you have a particular story transcending the results chapters? Or are they likely to be more isolated and/or separate? Remember, a thesis does not have to be chronological, so data you acquire at the end of your project can go at the start of your thesis and vice versa. This need not be a rigidly fixed plan, as things can (and do) change with new findings. Discuss how you see your thesis being structured with your supervisor and sketch out a list of figures that you want to include for each chapter – you may only be able to clearly do this for one of two (or none!) at the moment.

Once you have an agreed plan, it's time to assess exactly what state your data is currently in. Start by gathering that which you already have and ensure it's well organised and accessible. For typical experimental data, you want to be aiming for at least between two and four individual experiments, with a total of at least 6–8 subjects in a group, without which applying statistics will be challenging. Likewise, for clinical trials or patient observation studies your $n$ numbers might be orders of magnitude higher and you should know what you need in advance through power calculations or previous studies. Always highlight the experiments that need repeating and tick off those which are done and looking good.

Understandably, researchers want to keep pushing ahead and not look back. But it's advisable to repeat experiments and tidy things up sooner rather than later. Firstly, it will help build your bank of real thesis data which will provide you with confidence and reassurance that getting your PhD is achievable. Second, you risk forgetting or de-skilling in the experiment if it's a particular technique or if the study is conducted in collaboration with others, there's no guarantee they'll all still be here in a year's time. Third, you may find what initially looked like a promising avenue of research actually shows nothing with repeats – it's much better to discover this now and avoid spending months of experiments on what turns out to be a false lead.

## From preliminary to publishable data

'Preliminary data' is a useful phrase. Like a 'shield' or 'lightsabre', it provides researchers with a sense of security when discussing or sharing their findings. But preliminary work is not publishable and will not get you far in a 200 page or more thesis. The second year is the time to make the transition from preliminary to publishable – your aim is to not use the phrases 'preliminary data' and 'third year' in the same sentence.

As discussed already you need to get your repeats done. For example, in an experimental study, an *n* of 3 from one experiment is preliminary; while an *n* of 9 from three experiments is solid data. Apply statistics and ensure they're correct. If this isn't an area you have experience in, then consult a statistician (see Chapter 4). While you should draw confidence from a graph with stars of significance, they're 'par for the course' in published literature and theses. You need to do something different or novel. Drawing on your reading and experiments to date, is there an angle you could adopt that would make your findings stand out? Perhaps your results have led you to a new area, but will they form a good paper?

Thinking in this way might seem premature, but it's an essential test of your progress both in terms of your results and your scientific thinking to date. If you publish a paper from your results, there's no reason why this can't form all (or most) of a results chapter in your thesis. Aim high and get your thinking cap on. To publish a paper, you'll need a beginning, middle and end. The beginning could be background or validation data; for example, that your disease model works as expected or in a clinical study it could be the baseline demographics of your study population. Have you demonstrated or collected this already? If not, when do you expect to? The middle of a paper will contain the thrust of your results that support or refute your hypothesis. Maybe you're looking at a new cell for the first time in a disease model or monitoring patients after administering a new drug regime; either way you're going to need to flesh out the main finding with a series of figures (experiments) that support this from a range of angles. Finally, the end of the paper should ideally highlight why this is so important (or at least deserves publication). This could be showing clinical data to support an animal model or demonstrating the efficacy of a drug or regime on survival, adherence and so on. This 'ending' will vary in its persuasiveness and is usually what distinguishes where you can expect to have your results published. High-impact factor journals will want to see the broad importance of the findings and expect a lot of data focusing on this, more modest journals will be happy with you presenting your observations and (aside from some creative phrases in your discussion) will let readers decide or investigate the implications of your study in detail.

Now back to you. Looking at your data so far, is there a story or meaning? If so, can you discern a potential beginning and middle? What about the end? This latter point is important, as procedures or experiments that might give you the best bit of data might need a lot of preparation or clearance. Check as soon as possible whether your prospective studies can be performed under the licence/regulations you're working on, if they can't act fast – there's nothing worse than being unable to do *that* experiment.

## Supervising junior students

The choice of whether you supervise a junior student is often taken by your supervisor. It's not unheard of to arrive at your desk one morning and find waiting unannounced for you, the scientific equivalent of Paddington Bear: a young fresh faced medical or science undergraduate student who has maybe 8 weeks (yes…weeks!) to get data for their project. Your second year can often be perceived to be the best time for you to supervise more junior research students. In the first year, you're too busy finding your own feet and in the third year you're in a panic to get everything finished and don't have time.

If you have the option to contribute to the design of a student's project, choose something that you would be doing anyway, otherwise you'll be creating a lot of extra work for yourself. Keep it simple, if they are undergraduate students this is probably their first time in a real science laboratory, most of the techniques will be new to them. When the student starts, explain the background to the project and the aims and objectives of the work they will be undertaking in lay terms. This will help them understand why they are there, other than to get their degree. It will also be beneficial for you too, by ensuring you've spent time thinking about the best way to tell the story of your project.

While having a student is invariably seen as a burden by time pressed PhD students, it can also be seen as an asset. Supervision experience can be added to your CV and is relevant for future employment and fellowship applications down the line. In more immediate terms, the old adage of 'two heads are better than one' is often true, particularly in science. Encourage your student to participate in discussions and ask questions, we've all noticed a mistake in our own thinking when explaining something to a new arrival. If you train them up well in the lab, their project can become part of the wider experiments you're doing, which means an extra pair of hands to help out on the experiment day in the lab or clinic (make sure they have full health, safety and ethical clearance!). As your student becomes more familiar with the project, you will discuss your and their findings and other publications. These discussions may well help stimulate new ideas and directions for your project.

When you are working with the student remember that as well as teaching them about the specifics required to undertake their project, you should also be helping them develop an understanding of more general scientific principles. This includes scientific ethics, integrity and rigour; explain to them why each of the controls have been included within the experiment; show them how to keep a detailed and accurate lab book; and teach them why they can't simply disregard data that doesn't show what they want it to show.

Finally, encourage them to be a good lab citizen by including them on the roster for the preparation of general reagents, or giving them the honour of taking over your turn.

If the student's work is directly related to your project, then you obviously have a vested interest in their success. It is, however, important to remember to also give them space to flourish or fail. Teaching them the techniques they require and supervising them the first couple of times they do the experiment is fine, doing all their lab work for them is not okay. Similarly, you will probably be expected to read their write up and suggest corrections, but avoid rewriting it for them. Most importantly, do not tidy up after them. You have to start as you mean to go on, otherwise you will have a messy lab for the entire time they're with you.

Finally, while having a student can be an added challenge, they can be highly rewarding and lead to new friendships and collaborations in years to come. It's particularly helpful to offer exchanges to overseas students, who can become part of your international network.

## The end of Year 2 review/assessment

Most universities have a review process for students at the end of their second year. If not, you should institute one of your own. This checkpoint is to assess whether your project is on course and likely to be submitted on time. There are therefore two broad scenarios we'll cover regarding this checkpoint: it's going well and not so well.

If it's going well, good for you. This review presents an opportunity to road test your final thesis outline and projected plan for the third year. Does your proposed thesis make sense and sound convincing? Where are the stress points you need to reinforce? Can you realistically do this work in the time you have left? Like all things, prepare and discuss a fall back plan. Push your reviewers to highlight potential opportunities and pitfalls, discuss your publication ambitions or expectations, including any which you have already published or submitted. Can they also see a paper(s) in this work? If not, then ask why. If your project has proceeded well to date, this is a time to shake yourself out of any potential complacency and reach consensus on your third-year plan.

If your project has gone not so well to date, you'd be minded to take a different approach. Whether it's because your project doesn't make sense or isn't working, it's better to come clean than conceal and hide. If it's going badly, your supervisor may also be burdened with the anxiety of how this will turn around; your reviewers won't be. They are therefore a fresh pair of eyes, highly motivated to help bring perspective and impetus to a stalling project.

However harsh they may (occasionally) appear, nobody wants to downgrade/ fail/red flag a student. So, enlist their support from the opening; as, however uncomfortable, it's always better to pop the balloon yourself: (e.g. spoken)

*Today I'll be presenting data relating to my PhD on X, it's safe to say that despite some early success, this project has had a trying year and I look forward to drawing on the expertise and insight of my reviewers in this review and going forward.*

Outline the problems that you have encountered and the steps that you have taken to try and surmount them. Use the opportunity to get fresh perspective on the issues that you're facing – are there solutions you haven't considered? Is there additional experimental support they could offer or connect you too, for example, a new antibody or disease model? Check whether in their opinion your project is salvageable, though bear in mind that an awful lot of data can be generated in a short period of time when the experimental environment is conducive. However, if you're only just writing the licence for your main experiments, they're going to take a pretty dim view. At this point it's worth exploring what the damage control options are – such as an alternative project, downgrade and so on. Note, it is very rare for you to be in such a problematic position at 24 months, but better to be aware than not.

If your project is salvageable but somewhat in 'special measures', it's likely your reviewers will organise an interim review, perhaps 3 months later to see if you've managed to progress against your defined remedial work plan. This will not only give you another deadline to motivate and work towards, but will send a clear message to you and your supervisor that people are watching and it's time to deliver. If they don't offer you such a review, then organise it yourself. It's quite possible that your project isn't going as badly as you felt after all, in which case you want to get good instruction on your final year to come. Again, check whether your proposed experiments are feasible and what you can hope to generate and or publish from your results.

Finally, regardless of how you feel your project has progressed to date, the late stage review can be a very stressful experience. While your 'Transfer' is fairly low-key and you're not expected to have a lot of data, the pressure hikes up a year on. You may be required to write a report as well as deliver a presentation. The latter could be to just your reviewers or a whole department. If your project is going well, use the report to add to your thesis Introduction or provide a skeleton outline of your thesis. Alternatively, you could aim for a review article or use the writing in a publication you're working on. If it's going badly, this is an ideal chance to change trajectory, you're not the first and won't be the last: so *carpe* that *diem*…

## Conclusion

The second year of a PhD can be the most testing. You're balancing a rapid change in your competencies which is outstripped only by the demands on your time. Forging ahead and generating new data is important, but so is making sure that which you have is solid and reproducible. Junior students can add an additional burden. It's not uncommon during these periods to occasionally wonder why you ever thought doing a PhD was a good idea. We hereby outline a few common pitfalls associated with the second year.

## Common pitfalls

1. *'I've little solid data and will soon develop full-blown panic.'*
   This is a common feeling but with a sensible strategy it can be addressed. Panic in very small doses (called mild panic) can be helpful in motivating you. Full-blown panic is unhelpful and will stifle your judgement. Identify what data is solid and utilise the thought processes outlined above. What is the logical step for that data? If you're concerned that your experimental techniques are to blame, get someone else to watch or conduct it with you. Alternatively, run a quick calibration experiment with an obvious outcome and check you can still get the expected result.

2. *'I'm supervising two first-year PhDs, a Masters, two Bachelors and an A-level student.'*
   While supervising a junior student can be joyous, you are doing so primarily as an ambassador of your supervisor. Though it's considerate for them to involve you in the decision, this does not always occur. You're within your right to express a desire to be consulted when such choices regarding junior students are being made. You are well within your right to raise concerns directly with your supervisor (and others, if necessary) if you're finding these responsibilities overwhelming. If you don't speak up, your supervisor may be unaware there's a problem, even when they trip up on the school of children tailing you. Be clear and direct, your job is to research and conduct a PhD not to teach endlessly.

3. *'My publication ambitions evoke open laughter.'*
   Like most things worthwhile, science needs a bit of imagination. It's not uncommon for others to struggle to see your ideas, or how things link together; especially if your data is thin or non-existent. However, while you have a duty to meet checkpoints and come up with the results, it's not your fault if others can't see where you're heading (though it's worthwhile getting your supervisor on board). Don't be knocked back by hawkish post-docs, keep focused and believe in your ability – they'll have the chance to read it all in print one day…

4. *'I can't see this becoming a thesis.'*
   You're probably pretty good now at writing a 20-page report of some sort
   or the odd 40 slide presentation. But talking about hundreds of pages can
   induce nausea for some PhD students. This is not the time to worry, you
   may already have started writing your Introduction or perhaps you've got
   a results chapter or two nailed. Putting it all together is daunting, but so
   long as you're laying good foundations in your data, it will come together.
   Rome wasn't built in a day and they had a lot more than one PhD student
   working on it.

# Chapter 8    Presenting and publishing as a PhD student

*Ashton Barnett-Vanes[1] and Henry D.I. De'Ath[2]*

[1] MB-PhD Candidate, St George's, University of London and Imperial College London, UK

[2] Surgical Registrar and Honorary Clinical Lecturer, Wessex Deanery and Queen Mary, University of London, UK

## Background

The skills acquired while undertaking a PhD should enable you to become an independent researcher. One of these key skills is the art of academic communication, namely presentations and publications, which will raise your academic profile and strengthen your future grant and funding applications. They will augment your CV and make you a more attractive prospective supervisor or employer. Yet, as with any skill, they require attention to detail, application and perseverance. This can be particularly trying for PhD students, who are forging their own identity in a crowded intellectual space. The intention of this chapter is to give you guidance and insight into the opportunities and challenges faced in presenting and publishing during a PhD. Specifically, it covers some of the more awkward and less described *considerations* of academic communication, which more general books may omit, to assist your success in publishing and presenting your research.

## Presentations

### Why should you present?

Learning to talk about and explain your research (especially to non-experts) is an essential skill. Presentations serve as an opportunity to disseminate your latest findings. They'll often place you at conferences and other symposia relevant to your field, affording you the chance to network with fellow scientists and researchers. Importantly, presenting leads to immediate peer review on account of the questions and comments you receive from the audience.

*How to Complete a PhD in the Medical and Clinical Sciences*,
First Edition. Edited by Ashton Barnett-Vanes and Rachel Allen.
© 2018 John Wiley & Sons Ltd. Published 2018 by John Wiley & Sons Ltd.

**Table 8.1** Common presentation settings

| Setting | Regional/National/International | Peer Review | Abstract |
|---|---|---|---|
| Journal Club | Regional | | |
| Research Group/Lab | Regional | | |
| Regional (e.g. deanery) | Regional/National | ✓ | ✓ |
| Conferences/Societies | Regional/National/International | ✓ | ✓ |
| Research Milestones | Regional | | |
| Patient Groups | Regional/National | ✓ | |
| Ethics Meetings | Regional/National | ✓ | |
| PhD Viva | Regional | | |
| School Visits | Regional/National | | |
| Institutions (e.g. Royal Societies) | Regional/National | ✓ | |

Such comments can be helpful in formulating new ideas or exploring novel techniques relevant to your research, as well as discerning how much you do and don't know about your project. Finally, your PhD viva is a presentation, and one where you must speak about your research at length and in detail. The more practice and familiarity you have talking about your work the better: nobody escapes the viva.

**Common presentation scenarios**

During your research studies, you will be faced with many scenarios and opportunities to present your research (Table 8.1). Presentations can be daunting. Experience and practice makes them less so.

Critical appraisal is a fundamental skill required for a PhD and it necessitates practice and repeated application. Research and lab based groups have frequent meetings where you'll be expected to present. However, even when you're not speaking there's much you can learn from observing others. If you don't have a group journal club established in your department, then set one up. Regional meetings can be a useful opportunity to 'test run' your presentation skills to a smaller and less familiar group, before taking on national or international gatherings. Conferences are typically run by or in conjunction with academic societies. Join those relevant to your field early in your PhD as they'll email you with the dates of upcoming meetings and how to submit an abstract. Scientific journals also feature calls for abstracts and pertinent symposia. Your academic research milestones (such as 9- and 18-month progress checks) are crucial to your PhD progress, and an ability to talk clearly and confidently about your work will assist you in a favourable outcome. Other less common scenarios such as ethics meetings, patient groups, school visits or science fairs are excellent opportunities to learn to speak clearly and simply about your work. Non-specialist discussions frequently add fresh perspective to your research.

## How to present

### Abstract submission

First, you'll need to write a concise abstract with a clear aim. The bulk of this should be results. Your methodology needs to be precise and give a clear overview of how the study was undertaken. Study design, subjects, time frame and scientific methods are common inclusions. A detailed description of your statistical analyses is not usually required (unless your PhD is investigating a specific method) and a short line on the tests you applied will suffice. For results, include statistics and make sure the most important numbers are in. There is a bias towards positive results so try and include these if you have any. Conclusions should be brief and factual, don't overstate your findings or their importance. Try and submit the abstract well before the deadline and apply for prize sessions, since you have nothing to lose and potentially much to gain. Do not duplicate a presentation or poster unless the conference guidelines explicitly state this is acceptable.

### Oral presentations

Allow yourself ample time to write it. Don't be afraid to be visually bold; opposing colours with sharp contrast work well as an effective and clear format. When it comes to formatting your slides, less is often more. Keep creative pictures and illustrations to a minimum and avoid bizarre clip art or pictures of your pet. Remember, slides are prompts for the audience to scan while you talk. Judicious use of figures, tables and diagrams are encouraged. These must be well labelled and easy to follow.

Check your fonts and colours on large screens and from a distance; what looks good on your work computer may not translate well to a projector or big screen. Use animations judiciously, they can help when presenting diagrams with several components, but on the whole, can interfere with your flow, distract listeners and are prone to failure. We've all seen someone accidently skip half their presentation while zealously tapping through their animations.

It's important to read the meeting guidelines and keep to the length allocated. Let the time inform the amount of content you include – better under than over. Everyone has their own preference on length and slide usage: as a rule, 1–2 slides per minute of your presentation is sensible. Your aim in such short presentations is to leave the audience with a handful of important points. Overwhelming them with facts and results will undermine the impact of your address. Ask yourself, what is it you want the audience to take away from your lecture? Practice your presentation in front of others and learn your personal introduction. Avoid, however, reciting your slides by heart or reading from a page. Instead, use the slides as prompts and make sure you state a few clear points for each. It's common to talk quickly under pressure, so take a deep breath and slow down. Take special time and thought to rehearse presenting your tables and illustrations. Clumsy and confusing explanations of illustrated background data can knock your confidence early in the presentation. While an excellent Introduction and overview can give a boost, and set you up nicely.

On the day of your presentation load your talk on the platform you are going to speak on well before your allocated spot. Ensure your presentation is working properly without formatting errors or components missing. Have a copy of your presentation on another drive or online just in case. Arrive on time for your session and attend the entirety of it. It will enable you to identify the tone of the forum and mood of the audience. Position yourself within easy access to the stage, as a shuffling and embarrassing exiting strategy from your seat is an unnecessarily awkward start. Before you begin talking, it is common courtesy to acknowledge and thank the chair of the meeting or society they represent. When starting, don't go overboard and avoid flamboyance and arrogance. A little humour is permissible, if it comes fairly naturally, but contrived attempts to be funny can be painful to witness.

Predict questions to your presentation and practice the answers. Know the evidence behind your topic, including landmark studies that you should be able to quote or reference in the presentation. Be sure to understand their methodology and results in detail and appreciate any limitations, but be cautious in criticising other work as the authors may well be in the audience. You can sometimes guide questions by making reference to them in your talk: 'I'd be happy to talk further on this at the end', for example. If you don't know the answer to a question, do not make it up on the spot. This is almost always obvious and risks undermining your presentation and wider academic reputation. Remember to thank the chair and audience and any questioners. It's courteous to acknowledge your funders and colleagues/collaborators on the final slide.

## Poster presentations

Poster presentations are a different form of information dissemination. Typically, they can be more time consuming to formulate so write them early and again pay close attention to the guidelines: layout, size, colour and content. Once finished, print the poster well ahead of the meeting. Your department or funder may subsidise printing charges in part or full. Do not be one of the delegates sticking sheets of A4 together on the day. Format posters so they're readable at a distance. Avoid overcrowding and lengthy sentences or paragraphs by using simple bullet points and tables or illustrations. Use subheadings to signpost the reader's way around your poster and ease readability.

On the day, stay at your poster at your allocated time. People will take interest in your work and often ask probing questions. Once again this is an opportunity for networking. While poster presentations are often viewed as less prestigious than oral, their benefit is the close and continued dialogue you can have with other delegates about your work. Exchanges and discussion face to face can get to the nub of issues you might never cover in a Q&A after an oral talk. Moreover, delegates may be more comfortable exploring certain issues or opportunities with you out of earshot of the whole conference hall – so look sharp.

### General considerations for presentations

Be conscious of your conduct at a conference or meeting. You represent yourself and your department at all times. Dress smartly but comfortably and in line with the dress code. Consider the country and its weather and take appropriate accessories, for example, if it's monsoon season, take an umbrella. Avoid self-promotion and be respectful to other speakers and delegates. It takes effort, hard work and some courage to present your work. Be wary of company representatives asking you to sign things. Finally enjoy yourself but maintain professionalism – you use the free bar at your own risk.

## Publications

There are several reasons to publish your work. From a researcher perspective, publishing results is the key contribution one can make to their research field. For your career, publications inform collaborators, funders or employers of your capacity to generate output. Finally, to be awarded a doctorate, your 3 years of research will need to have generated at least three chapters of peer review quality original research. Submitting a bound thesis in which some or all the content has been published will serve as tangible evidence to examiners that you have achieved this goal. Indeed, certain universities permit you to bind your published papers together as a thesis, while others (including continental Europe and North East Asia) may mandate the publication of two or three papers before you can even qualify for thesis submission.

Through submitting a paper you'll receive peer review. Even when faced with rejection, the comments and observations you receive can improve your work and highlight areas you need to address. It is better to know these prior to viva day. Beware that writing a paper takes a sustained period of time, and the journey from submission to publication is equally lengthy. You should anticipate several months before your work is in print, particularly if you've had rounds of revision or rejection (covered below). Whole books in this series and others have covered the ins and outs of writing a paper[1]. In this section, we'll cover a breadth of issues pertinent to a PhD student, and provide details and guidance on the two most common articles you'll publish: an original research article and a review article.

In considering to write a paper from your research you should follow the three Ws: why, what and where.

## Why?

This first question to ask yourself is why are you trying to publish? Do you have a method that deserves dissemination? Perhaps a novel positive or negative finding that furthers understanding? Whatever the reason, make sure you have one. If you can't justify to yourself why you're writing a paper, convincing readers in print will be impossible. Your paper must have a narrative.

## What?

Having convinced yourself and supervisor of the merits of writing the article, you now need to decide what will go in it. Without doubt, you'll have a centre-piece section of data – the most significant results to the *story*. But this needs to be supported by a strong foundation of findings or validation. Information overload is of no help, and while the highest impact factor journals require substantive amounts of manuscript and supplemental data, typically six well-chosen and presented figures should suffice for most respectable journals.

## Where

Once you've decided on the data, it's time to look at where you intend to submit it. This might seem premature given you've only just decided on the figures to include; however, journals have highly diverse procedures for content presentation and writing. You want to know close to the outset how the article might need to be written. Your supervisor should have a good idea of what kind of journal and impact factor to aim for. Inform this discussion by checking the journal rankings for your field, paying attention to both impact factor and the quartile ranking. Websites such as SCImago or ThomsonReuters rankings can assist in this process.

## Writing an original research article

### Overview

Now you're set on the reasons for writing your paper, have decided upon the data to include and identified your target journal(s), it's time to start writing. While everyone has a slightly different way of writing their papers, we'll outline a simple and reliable method to get you from A to P. Bear in mind that your results will inform the whole paper so get your figures in order first (see later). With your figures done, focus next on the Introduction, results and discussion. Whilst everyone differs, sections such as the abstract, methods and conclusions can be left until later in your article preparation. To make things easier we've presented each in the order they'll typically appear in the finished product.

## Title

Choosing a title can be harder than it sounds and it's not uncommon for it to change several times over the course of writing. Alongside a main title, most journals ask for a short or running title of perhaps 5–10 words (or around 45 characters). If you're struggling, start with this condensed version and expand it slightly. At a minimum, the title should detail the main finding, model or intervention and type of subjects involved.

For example, which of the two below better informs you as a prospective reader?

1. Neutrophils respond to circulating LPS through a TLR-dependent mechanism in a human model of septic shock
2. Investigation of the immune response to LPS: a role for TLRs
   (The answer is 1.)

A short running title could be: 'Neutrophils and TLR's in LPS human septic shock'.

## Abstract

These are usually 250–300 words in length. 'Introduction', 'Methods', 'Results' and 'Conclusions' are typical subheadings but check as some journals alter their format. The abstract should be able to stand alone online and there is good evidence to suggest it is used to inform whether people cite your work. It should therefore be written to entice the reader to read the full paper, while also accurately informing them of the study design, purpose and main findings.

## Introduction

This should set the scene for your reader. Keep it brief, but ensure it is rich in background, evidence and, towards the end, persuasive argument. On completion of the Introduction, the reader should be convinced of the necessity of your paper and persuaded by its aims. It's customary for you to briefly state in the last sentence what you did or found as a preview to the research you will present; however, this may be omitted depending on the journal. State your aims clearly at the end of the Introduction. Ensure these aims match the narrative of your paper. Two sentences will suffice, as you will have further chance later on to contextualise your work.

## Methods (and materials)

Your methods are where you prove your work to be valid. Technically, your Methods section should be written such that another group or individual given the same materials could replicate your study and its findings. Be precise, detailed and start with the obvious factors like study subjects and ethical approval. Describe the study type, experimental design, setting and if necessary, duration. Explain recruitment criteria if appropriate. List the samples you collected and interventions made including their timepoints. Describe the techniques or instruments used, citing previous studies where necessary. List the name, dosage and route of administration for drugs. Write the company/provider and country it's headquartered in whenever you mention a new material. If using multiple reagents like antibodies it might be easier for you and the reader to present their details in an orderly table. Include antibody clone, where you purchased it, the dilution used and it's fluorochrome. Towards the end of your methods you should include a description of the data analysis and statistical methods employed including the programme used. Many journals will get a statistician to review your work; incorrect use or interpretation of your stats will result in rejection, or at best a request for revision.

## Results

As discussed earlier, your results are the make or break of your paper. It's typical for figures to build in detail and significance sequentially. Early figures might be baseline data from your study group, while latter figures might show novel observations or mechanistic data. Present and describe your results chronologically in the text, starting with Figure 1A onwards. You may be required to detail the statistics of key findings in the text alongside qualitative descriptions, but again this is journal specific. Ensure you avoid wider interpretation of your results and keep the style consistent, for example, 'Fig' or 'Figure', $p < 0.05$ or $p = 0.04$, not both. Resist the temptation to statistically overanalyse the data. If something is obviously not different between groups, putting an 'ns' for non-significant on the figure is unnecessary.

Your figures need to look professional and fit the journal requirements. Typical software packages like Microsoft Excel, GraphPad Prism or SPSS enable simple graph or table drawing. Maximise their utility and appearance by importing these images into professional artwork packages like Adobe Illustrator or Photoshop. Factors to look out for include the type of image file (TIF, PNG or JPEG), the colour scheme (RGB or CMYK) and compression/size. Failure to adhere to journal guidance will result in endless technical revisions and corrections before your paper is even sent out for review.

## Discussion

In the discussion, your aim is to ensure your readers understand not only what you have shown, but also the relevance and implications of your findings. Begin with a general summary of what you have presented. Then interpret your results and place them in the context of the wider literature by citing relevant articles. You have greater flexibility to cover data in the order you choose in this section, but make sure it is easy to follow and flows logically. Examine the potential significance of your findings and their clinical or experimental implications. Towards the end of the discussion, recognise and state the limitations of your work. Touch on areas of future work and attempt to frame the next investigations; however, avoid detailed description of future studies as this is beyond the remit of an original research article. Complete the discussion with a brief conclusion and avoid the 'further research is required' line.

## Conclusion

This should serve as a succinct summary of your work and conclude with the final take home message. It's worth writing this when your discussion is finalised. A good conclusion should feel reinforcing, not repetitive, and must not state anything that hasn't already been presented and discussed robustly in the preceding sections.

## Bibliography

Chapter 5 covers ways to create citations and bibliographies in detail. Using a citation management software is *strongly* advised and many will enable you to generate journal specific bibliographies that are fully formatted.

# Writing a review article

## Overview

Review articles, whether *narrative* or *systematic*, have long been seen as the purview of established researchers and academics with track records in a selected field. This is particularly true of narrative reviews, which are either solicited by journal editors or only otherwise considered if authors have demonstrable track records. Systematic reviews and meta-analyses, however, are increasingly open for researchers of any level to perform so long as they are done well. As a PhD student, there are four common situations in which you could write a review article for peer-reviewed publication:

1. After your Year 1 transfer or Year 2 review (see Chapters 5 and 7, respectively).
2. As a required component of submitting an original research article.
3. During or after the writing of your thesis.
4. Because your supervisor has been invited to write one.

## Systematic reviews: The basics

A systematic review seeks to examine and describe original research data in a clearly defined and transparent way. In the first instance, you'll need to define exactly what you're seeking to review with your co-authors. Two obvious opportunities where you should consider writing a systematic review are during your transfer and when writing up your PhD.

For the transfer report, you'll be required to provide a literature review on your PhD area. Given a PhD should be novel in some way, this can provide an opportunity to perform a systematic review for the transfer report which you can go on to publish. It's wise to get the early approval of your supervisor on this, as once you begin the review you can't change the search terms or inclusion/exclusion criteria (without re-doing the whole process). As covered earlier in this chapter, be prudent in identifying target journals and consider corresponding in advance with the Editor on their potential interest. Usually your supervisor/senior author might be better placed to perform this for you. Between submitting your transfer report and thesis, at least 2 years would have passed. There's likely to be new papers and understanding in your field, including (fingers crossed!) those you've published yourself. The Introduction to your thesis will include a summary of the literature in your field, again presenting an opportunity to perform a systematic review. Other opportunities will be if submitting an original paper to a very high impact journal, for example, *The Lancet* (among others) have begun to ask authors of original papers to add a short systematic review component to their article, to better contextualise the significance of their work. Finally, you might find yourself writing a systematic review you'd never intended to if your supervisor is invited to contribute one. Naturally, this is an opportunity to be seized.

Alongside systematic reviews, a meta-analysis might also be indicated. These studies seek to examine the results of particularly focused research, including an analysis of their significance or impact, and are particularly useful for interventional studies such as clinical trials. If your PhD is looking at the efficacy or potential of a new drug or diagnostic test, a review and meta-analysis of existing studies would be wise, either at the start, transfer stage, or during the writing up of your PhD.

## Introduction

Keep the Introduction rich but concise and outline why a review is needed. It's important to highlight the existing literature in passing, but save the detail for later in the paper. If there are previous reviews in this area explain why another is needed, for example was it done decades ago? If so, what might have changed since?

## Methods

You'll need to be very detailed in describing what data sources you searched, and include the strategy you employed. Did you use a specific search interface such as Ovid SP? Ensure you describe the inclusion/exclusion criteria; the dates over which the review took place; restrictions placed on the review such as language or date of publication. It's highly advisable to look at the PRISMA guidelines on systematic reviews in advance[1]. Describe who reviewed the studies for inclusion or exclusion, which data points you extracted and how.

## Results

Your first figure should typically detail the results of your search strategy. A flow diagram is particularly sensible, allowing you to illustrate how many articles were excluded and for what purpose. At the end of the diagram detail the study characteristics and provide a table on the study population with information such as: when and where the articles were published, number of participants, study design, interventions trialled (if applicable) and so on. Describe the main sections of these studies in subheadings. As in original articles, avoid interpreting the results at this stage but describe the details in full including statistics used.

## Discussion and conclusion

This is the chance to bring the studies included in your review together and present a coherent synthesis of their findings to date. At this stage, it's important to appraise the quality of other studies as well as their findings. This necessitates you paying significant attention to detail in the methods and results of the papers included. If there are important details missing or components of the study which weren't performed correctly, make this clear. In concluding, you may choose to provide a proposal or recommended framework on future studies (but don't get carried away).

## Narrative reviews

If during your PhD you're able to publish several original articles, you and your supervisor could have a strong case to write a narrative review in an established journal. Alternatively, this may be a review your supervisor is invited to perform. Either way, narrative reviews often afford authors greater flexibility than systematic reviews, including the chance to put forward their own creative take on the field, such as diagrammatic figures on scientific mechanisms or proposed hypotheses. If well written and in a reputable journal, such reviews can accrue citations for years to come, bringing prestige for you and co-authors.

## Final steps

### Covering letter

Most journals will require you to submit a covering letter with your paper. This should be brief (two short paragraphs will suffice), explaining your article and why it's important. Ensure you get the Editor's name and credentials correct.

## Acknowledgements

It's good practice to acknowledge help and support where you have received it. For example, histology, imaging or flow cytometry technicians would be courteous to acknowledge. Funders may also be detailed here, though this will vary depending on the journal.

## Writing style

Look at published articles to be familiar with the writing style. Write in the past tense. Quality of your written English is important. Short sentences, good punctuation and correct spelling are needed for easy reading and will be expected by reviewers. Both your institution and the journal can help with language services if English is not your first language. Be cautious when using common words with specific scientific meanings, for example confusing prevalence with incidence. Check the journal policy regarding abbreviations, which should be used judiciously.

## Managing the process

Despite research being your reason to exist as a PhD student, publishing scientific research can be slow, daunting and at times a thankless task. Here's some key hurdles to keep an eye on from the outset.

## Authors

Deciding who is going to be an author and in what order they will feature on the paper is crucial. This is a decision to be taken with your supervisor early on. If you have undertaken the majority of the research and written the paper to be published, then you must be first author. This is not just fair, but an ethical requirement (see the ICMJE[2] for further details). It is typical for your main supervisor to be last author, and together these are the two most coveted positions on a paper. If you have equally done the same amount of work as someone else you can be joint first authors, often denoted on the manuscript by the line 'both authors contributed equally to this manuscript'. However, note that only one of your names will be first on PubMed and so on. Ensure authors are aware from the outset of their involvement with the paper and have agreed to their position; there are endless horror stories involving people who've disagreed with author position, which can sometimes be the difference between a grant or good REF score or not. Be aware that some journals limit the number of authors that can be involved. The corresponding author is the person for which all journal correspondences are directed, and all reader queries post-publication. However, this person can change between submission and publication, so it's advisable to name yourself (if first author) as the correspondent for journal communication, as you're likely to be less busy responding to journal queries than senior colleagues or supervisors. After acceptance, journals permit the corresponding author to be revised. It's common for you to need to circulate an author agreement or competing interest disclosure form to your co-authors and chase up responses.

### Drafts

Communicating with your authors and getting their input on your article draft is an ethical requirement. However, be strategic about it. There's no point sending something out repeatedly for minor corrections from 10 different authors. First, get their agreement on the main contents (e.g. figures), then write the paper and revise it with key authors (e.g. your supervisor) before sharing a well-developed and vetted draft with other co-authors. Be mindful of their own workloads and holiday periods in returning annotated drafts. Ensure too, that you're keeping track of these drafts with well labelled and stored file names.

### Open access and your thesis

Many journals offer open access options to authors, while some journals are solely open access such as the *PLoS* and *BMJ* Group *Open* series. Check in advance if your institution has funds to support open access publishing. This is particularly important when considering your thesis. If you intend to publish work from your research that will be included in your thesis prior to its submission, you need to check carefully on the open access arrangements. As it stands, including your journal-published figures in your thesis requires specific licensing agreements to be in place, which are commonly covered by open access publishing licences. Discuss this matter with your institutional library and the journal in advance, as often the open access decision is not made until after paper acceptance.

### Journal amendments and response to reviewer comments

It's common for reviewers to recommend revisions to your article before final acceptance. It's important to accommodate these requests. Though unlikely, don't let these distort or change key components of your paper without good reason. If the journal has asked for amendments perform these promptly as it suggests they're willing to publish your paper. Answer and acknowledge each point made by the reviewers on a separate page, and track the changes you make to the manuscript. Make sure the separate letter describes the changes and highlights where they can be found in your manuscript. Should your paper be rejected, in most cases this will be final. However, if you feel this is unwarranted you can email the Editor and appeal the rejection, which on occasion may be successful if clearly justified.

## Other considerations

### Peer reviewing

In time, you may be asked by a journal to peer review a paper. This is flattering, and good both for your critical appraisal skills and CV. Be cautious of the extra burden of work and avoid unheard of 'vulture' journals with poor reputations. Decline to review papers outside your knowledge and experience, and always be respectful of other people's work and the effort they have made. Be balanced in your critique and punctual with your responses. Journals are increasingly performing 'open peer review' and publishing reviewer comments with the final manuscript. While not uncommon, do not peer review a paper if you have a relationship with the author or you strongly suspect the anonymised author is a friend or colleague. However informal the understanding, it's unethical to do so and could haunt your reputation years down the line.

## Conclusion

Presenting and publishing is a central component of the PhD journey. While early stage PhD students may feel ill-equipped to write a research article, this should be in the back of your mind as the eventual goal. Whether presenting or publishing, follow the preparation and submission rules. Finally, PhD students shouldn't need to navigate the associated challenges of publishing alone; ask your supervisor or mentor for help in selecting the target journals and building your co-author list.

## References

1. Hall, G. *How to Write a Paper*. Wiley-Blackwell, 2012.
2. Preferred Reporting Items for Systematic Reviews and Meta-Analyses (PRISMA) website, www.prisma-statement.org/(accessed 8 December, 2016).

## Further reading

1. ICMJE, Defining the role of authors and contributors. Available online at: www.icmje.org/recommendations/browse/roles-and-responsibilities/defining-the-role-of-authors-and-contributors.html, 2016. (accessed 8 December, 2016).

## Chapter 9  Landing and writing up: Year 3

*Manu Chhabra[1] and E. Allison Green[2]*

[1] Doctor, National University Hospital, Singapore and University of Cambridge, Singapore, UK

[2] Senior Lecturer, University of York, UK

### Background

Most students enter their final year with a sense of relief – and at the same time – in a state of sheer panic. On the one hand, the hard grind at the lab bench or in the clinic is almost over; on the other, fear creeps in as to whether you've got enough data for a thesis that might appear the length of *War and Peace*. Take heart, you will get through it. By the time you enter the final year, you will have (perhaps subconsciously) honed your self-belief, tenacity and intellectual knowledge; all attributes that you'll need to get to the finish line. In this chapter, we'll focus on your final research year and how to efficiently write a great PhD thesis.

### An exit strategy

The final year of research is almost always the most productive. This is primarily because of the foundations you've laid in preceding years, optimising your experiments and problem solving. In the final year, the project should become increasingly focused, with set goals to achieve based on your finalised hypothesis. At the start of this year it's essential to have a protracted meeting with your supervisor(s), where your year plan evolves and is agreed. This meeting will serve many purposes, one of the most important is to review your current data and critically assess its strengths and weaknesses, Box 9.1 has some key questions to ask yourself.

If the answer is 'no' to any of these questions, consider whether you have the time and resources available to address them. This may involve setting up collaborations with others in your field to help complete a few key

*How to Complete a PhD in the Medical and Clinical Sciences,*
First Edition. Edited by Ashton Barnett-Vanes and Rachel Allen.
© 2018 John Wiley & Sons Ltd. Published 2018 by John Wiley & Sons Ltd.

> **Box 9.1** What to ask yourself before a final year meeting
>
> - Have you considered all the caveats (alternative explanations for your data as opposed to being dogmatic in interpretation so it fits your hypothesis)?
> - Do you have all the appropriate controls in your experiments to validate your data?
> - Do have the necessary statistical power to confirm the significance of your data?
> - Is the hypothesis focused and your data supportive of it?

experiments or attain resources you need. Your supervisor will be invaluable in this regard. Additionally, you need to decide upon a timeline for completing your experimental work – not as easy as it sounds. There'll always be one more experiment to do, one more result that will make the data even better, one more…STOP! Decide and stick to the date you stand down. There are instances when supervisors have had to hide pipettes or even remove lab access from their students, in order to get them to write up; be warned and go willingly.

## The X Factor results

As you approach the middle of your final year, it's time to consider winding down lab operations and focusing on your thesis write up. But before you can start writing, you need to know which data to include in your thesis. While it's advisable to continuously appraise and analyse your data as you go, it's easy to slip into full experimental mode and let it pile up, especially as time or money begins to run out. But whether a mountain or mole-hill, you've got to get to grips with all your data before you put finger to keyboard. Thoroughly analyse, assort and label it so it's easy to access and draw upon repeatedly during your writing up. It may be necessary to reanalyse old data too, given you might know things now you didn't then. Either way, after this process you should be in a position to write, clear in the knowledge that you're aware of all the data you have.

A thesis will usually contain 3–5 chapters of research. Depending on the style of your data, this will vary significantly in size and form. One thing will remain, however; examiners do not want to be bored or buried by your thesis: yes, size does matter. Now fully analysed, you're looking for data that convincingly supports or refutes your thesis – this is 'X Factor' data, but avoid reams of pages of inconsequential data that do not have any discernible relationship to your main research narrative – this is Z factor data, you know, for Zzzz… Knock out some rough figures and agree with your supervisor on the data you're going to include. We'll cover the writing of your results later in this chapter.

## Before you start writing

Firstly, well done on completing your research. It may seem, surveying your accumulated data that the hard work is over but don't underestimate the challenge of incorporating it into a concise, informative and grammatically correct scientific thesis. The thesis is not a research paper, it's a piece of scientific writing that documents your skill sets of unbiased review of scientific literature, critical thinking and analysis, and communication. This is your 'introduction' to your viva examiners and the quality of the thesis will dictate the line of questioning you'll experience during your viva. For example, a poorly put together methods section will raise doubts in an examiner's mind that you performed the experiments. Likewise, introductions and discussions that seem haphazard with limited flow yet an excellent results section will flag up whether you had an up to date understanding of your research field or whether you actually wrote the whole thesis yourself. A strong scientific thesis is critical for completing your PhD. In the following sections, we will discuss the requirements to produce such a thesis based on our experience as PhD candidates and examiners.

One of the most important aspects of writing a thesis is to familiarise yourself with the guidelines for thesis submission by your university. Thus, before you start writing make note of:

- *Departmental and external deadlines*: This can include pre-submission approval or an 'intention to submit' form that needs to be submitted in sufficient notice prior to the actual submission. Signatures from various individuals may be needed so contact in advance and be mindful of their vacations.
- *Preferred formatting guidelines*: Your university will have outlined the preferred font type and size as well as line spacing preferences and the size of the margins (both for submission and binding). In general, there is a maximum word count, this may or may not include references and figure legends, so do check carefully. Similarly, make sure you comply with the preferred format for figures/tables/page numbering, large genomic data sets and references. Keep in mind that your thesis will be read by examiners who have high workloads; after which it will be in the public domain, where universities have an obligation to ensure it's accessible to a broad range of readers.
- *Requirements for an embargo on the thesis*: As mentioned before, the thesis once complete will be in the public domain. Theses should contain publishable data, and in general, research journals will not accept data that has been previously published (with the exception of conference abstracts). If your thesis contains data you envisage publishing in a research paper it's essential you place it under embargo for a period of time, during which you can submit and publish your articles.

Good communication and feedback from your supervisor is one of the most important aspects for writing a thesis. It's vital you arrange a meeting with your supervisor at the start of the write up to explore the draft structure of your thesis, timelines for completing subsections (Introduction, methods, results, discussion) and your supervisor's availability for the duration of the write up. In general, it can take anywhere between 2 and 5 months to write a PhD thesis. It's advisable to give your supervisor defined subsections, rather than a whole draft for rapid feedback; not only are they unlikely to have time to read a whole thesis carefully and quickly, but the initial constructive feedback on your quality of writing will motivate you and set the standards for the rest of the thesis. Do not aim for perfection prior to giving your supervisor your initial writings, they're fully aware a draft is a 'work in progress'.

Lastly, it is important that you identify a good location where you feel you can write your thesis in a quiet and focused manner. Some departments might have areas to write, but you could be easily distracted. The library could be a good alternative. Writing up at home is another option. Here, the benefit is you can potentially cut down on accommodation costs for a couple of months, banking any stipend you have remaining. On the downside, the personal space you have available to relax and 'switch-off' might feel diminished. If considering writing at home, beware there can be a *form* for that. Finally, it's possible to use different locations to write different sections of your thesis depending on what they need. For example, in writing the results section you might benefit from close proximity to your supervisor; while reviewing literature for the Introduction may need the studious silence of a library or bedroom. Figure out what works for you and stick to it.

## Writing your thesis: Part 1

Theses have a defined structure, and guidelines will be available from your department or postgraduate research office. An example structure is used throughout the rest of this chapter. In general, the first few pages will be devoted to the declaration that the thesis is your own work, list of abbreviations used in the thesis, Table of Contents, list of figures/tables and Acknowledgements. Thereafter, the main body of the thesis will be chapters devoted to the thesis: Abstract, Introduction, Materials and Methods, Results, Discussion, Conclusion, along with Future Work and finally the Bibliography. The order in which you write each of these sections is entirely up to you. Some students prefer to start by putting together their material and methods chapter, which is by far the least intellectually challenging and can boost student confidence to see 'words on paper'. Others start with the results section as it's the chapter that will shape the rest of the thesis, and is therefore the most challenging and time consuming. It's recommended that you start with the results; however, irrespective of where you start, stick to finishing that chapter and don't jump from one to another – it can be demoralising to see reams of scattered and unfinished content.

## Declaration

The declaration is a legal statement that the research performed and the writing of the thesis is the work of the student submitting. The wording of the declaration is usually standard and provided by the student's postgraduate office. Some universities require the declaration to be signed by the student and co-signed by their supervisor. It's possible that some aspects of your research may incorporate unpublished data from a collaborator or required technical input/collaboration from a colleague. Don't worry about that. It's acceptable to submit a thesis where a small amount of the work was conducted by others, or where large amounts were generated in collaborative research settings – so long as these individuals are properly acknowledged for their contributions and the majority of the work is your own to defend.

## Abbreviations

Theses have a list of abbreviations used throughout that serves as a quick reference guide for the reader to refresh their memory. You can keep building this throughout your thesis or it can be easily generated by doing the following: at the use of each new word or phrase you wish to abbreviate – typically those which you'll use repetitively – enclose it in quote marks, for example, flow cytometry ('FCM'). At the end of your thesis, use the search function in your word processer to find the bracket-quotation mark (', so long as you haven't enclosed any other words in this, you'll be able to copy each of these abbreviations and their full phrase into a computer spreadsheet, sort them alphabetically and copy the typeset list back into your thesis document.

## Acknowledgements

The awarding of a PhD is not just a reflection of your critical thinking and analysis skills or your ability to communicate scientific research to a wide community; it's also a measure of your professionalism. Examiners do read Acknowledgements and can bring students to task in the viva if they feel the student has, without true justification, been dismissive of the input from their supervisor and/or colleagues. The set of people you wish to acknowledge is entirely your choice, but in general: supervisors, laboratory colleagues, collaborators, friends and family tend to be acknowledged, with a short explanation of their contributions. Do remember to acknowledge the funder(s) of your PhD. Acknowledgements can be funny, witty and show your sense of humour, so long as they're respectful and do not violate university policy!

## Table of Contents, figures and tables

The Table of Contents (ToC) is your major reference index for the thesis and helps examiners understand and follow the structure of your thesis. You'll also be expected to provide a list of figures and a list of tables. There are two ways to do this: the extremely long and painful way (copy and pasting at the end); or the simple and efficient way – albeit prone to the odd technical meltdown. We'll cover the latter here using Microsoft Word as an example, though all good word processors can do this.

Throughout your thesis writing, it's essential to use the styles function to give your thesis a hierarchical heading structure. Say you have four levels: Chapter title > Chapter section > Chapter heading > Chapter sub-heading.

Using styles, you can format these headings in their appearance and size, and create customisable ToCs including as many or as few layers, for example:

1.      Introduction

1.1     Innate immunity

1.1.1   NK cells

1.1.1.1 NK cell development

If you decide to move headings around or change something after revisions from your supervisor, using styles will permit you to rearrange the ToC in one click. The same principle applies to figures and tables. In Word, this is performed via the 'Caption' toolbar. A figure or table caption will ascribe it a number or letter (e.g. Figure 2.4) depending on the chapter you are in (using styles) or your own numerical preference, and again will allow you to easily create a list (effectively a ToC) of tables or figures. As before, this will update depending on whether you move your figures or tables around or delete them. Additionally, by using the 'cross-reference' function, you can refer to the figure or table in the text of your thesis, and this too keeps updated depending on the status and order of your figures. So, if you have written your whole thesis, and then decide to move one figure, the copy-and-paste approach would require renumbering of all the figures and in-text references to account for the new order (the very thought can induce palpitations). However, if you have used the cross-reference function for your in-text references to a figure, this will update to the new figure order automatically, saving you traumatically boring hours of corrections, and avoiding the real risk of a mistake that undermines your whole thesis. Further guidance and resources are included at the end of this chapter – it's highly recommend you take the time to become competent with this function at the outset of your writing.

## Bibliography

As discussed in Chapter 5, use of a citation manager is essential for writing a thesis. The style of the bibliography will depend on your university guidance. As citation managers can be prone to unbelievable bouts of meltdown, regularly check your citation placeholders are functioning and correct errors as they arise.

Check if your university has guidelines on how your pages should be numbered, some students prefer to use roman numerals for numbering the pages preceding the main text; however, so long as the ToC is clear, the style of numbering is usually at the discretion of the student.

## Writing your thesis: Part 2

Like most scientific writing, the objective of a thesis is to create a 'flow' of information. Each subsection of a chapter should build on the information from the previous subsection – this is called 'spiral' writing; and will ensure by the time the examiner/reader reaches the end of the chapter, they comprehend the major points you wish to make and appreciate their significance.

---

*Top tip*

Use two or more computer monitors to boost your efficiency at writing and cross-referencing your thesis.

---

## Introduction

The Introduction enables you to review the scientific field your thesis is related to; however, this 'review' is not to be mistaken for a 'Discussion', see Box 9.2 for an example.

Historically, theses tend to have one major Introduction that builds from basic information on the thesis subject matter, to a focused in-depth review of the area of research the project tackles. Increasingly, this Introduction is being supplemented by introductions to each results chapter. Thus, while the main Introduction chapter used to be long, expansive and highly detailed; today this is often more condensed (e.g. 50 pages double spaced); with short 4–6 page introductions at the start of each results chapter that are more detailed and focus on setting the scene for the data to be presented.

---

**Box 9.2** Spot the difference – Introduction versus Discussion

- A student's thesis is focused on analysing the efficacy of rituximab therapy on ameliorating type 1 diabetes, and the rationale for using the therapy is based on the role of B cells (the target cell for rituximab) in the autoimmune condition. In the Introduction, you would write, 'B cells have been shown to play a critical role in type 1 diabetes progression [Serreze et al.]'.
- However, as a discussion point, you would clarify the statement by critiquing what Serreze et al. actually showed in their manuscript to prove the role of B cells in type 1 diabetes, for example, 'B cells have been shown to play a critical role in type 1 diabetes progression'. For example, Serreze et al., using a murine strain devoid of B cells documented an inability to induce spontaneous type 1 diabetes with respect to B cell sufficient murine strains'.

---

Whichever approach you wish to take for writing an Introduction, inevitably there will be a large body of literature to review. Deciding on the scope of the literature review is a daunting task, so bullet point all your main findings and ask yourself 'What background information would a person need to have to understand why I performed this series of experiments and the significance of the results?'. By doing this you will start to identify the information essential to understanding the rationale for the research questions you posed; this is your 'need to know' information and should be reviewed in some depth. In addition, your thesis should demonstrate knowledge of the general field of your research topic, including points that are slightly tangential to your research hypotheses. If you don't demonstrate the breadth of your understanding now, you're inviting your examiner to grill you on it during the viva; but don't go overboard, keep additional information concise. The last paragraph in any Introduction will always be focused on the unmet need of your research field. This should contextualise the aims and hypothesis that follow immediately thereafter.

## Aims and Hypothesis

Your Hypothesis will normally be a few sentences, and your main project aims (~3–5) should be written as bullet points. Write your project aims after completing your results section so they align perfectly. Remember, science is dynamic and your initial aims may have been superseded by the data you accumulated, as well as the research field in general, over the past three years.

## Materials and Methods

This is the easiest chapter to write as you are simply documenting how you performed experiments; however, as simple as this chapter may seem, remember that the examiner needs to be convinced you performed the

**Box 9.3** Materials and Methods checklist

- Names and suppliers of reagents and specialist equipment
- Names of software packages used
- Names of cell-line and antibody clones (this is usually best tabulated)
- Composition of specialised solutions made in-house
- Animal strains and their sources
- Ethical approval for studies undertaken (animal and/or clinical)

experiments – any researcher should be able to replicate your findings from the methodology detailed. You'll also need to document what materials you used and where they originated from, that is, a company, collaborator or in-house. See Box 9.3 for an example checklist of points to include.

If you use a commercially available kit, do not make the mistake of stating you used 3 μL of the 'red cap tube' – state what reagent is in the tube. If the company does not provide that information, it is acceptable to state you used this kit 'according to the manufacturer's instructions'.

Methods, like all chapters, have subsections to create focus and clarity. Here are a few examples:

1. Animals/patients – document all the strains used, sources and ethical approval to conduct experiments; or your recruitment criteria, setting and ethical clearance.
2. Cell preparations – document how you prepared cells from, for example, spleen, versus lymph nodes.
3. DNA/RNA preparation – document exactly how you prepared DNA/ RNA from your cells.

Note, you do not have to repeat how the cells were isolated, as you tackled that in the previous section.

## Results

As mentioned previously, the results section is usually the most time-consuming chapter to write. This chapter tests your critical thinking and communication skills; not only do you need good judgement on what data to show, but you also need to deliver it in a clear, informative and logical way. Designing a good figure that displays complex data in an accessible manner is a lengthy process often requiring countless iterations, and should therefore be started as soon as possible after deciding upon your final data.

### Selection and ordering of data

As discussed earlier, you should now be aware of all the data you have available. One decision you need to make early, is what data to present as figures and what can be classified as 'data not shown'. This will be informed by your research narrative. Like any good crime/mystery case, a scientific project follows a similar pattern; you have an event (a hypothesis that tackles an unmet need in your research field) and a resolution (your keynote result that resolves your hypothesis). Along the way, you accumulate a series of experimental data that builds support for your keynote result; this experimental pathway will include 'negative' data that disproves – and 'positive' data that supports – the rationales you make as you progress towards the keynote result. Remember that a thesis is not a research paper, and so does not have space limitations sometimes seen in journals that restrict you to focusing on positive results. Moreover, a thesis full of 'data not shown' could precipitate concern among examiners and lead to a grilling at your viva.

Don't feel under pressure to avoid data that didn't work out. Occasionally, whole results chapters (in multi-chapter theses) can be dedicated to a technique or method that ultimately did not work. This showcases to examiners your ability to critically think and problem solve – key features expected of a graduating PhD candidate. Data which is relevant but not central to your research, such as optimising data can be cited as 'data not shown' or included as 'supplementary' information in an appendix at the end of your thesis.

Remember, usually there are multiple results chapters; if you used multiple approaches in your thesis for example, generation of genetic constructs, immunisation with these novel genetic constructs and translation of the therapy to humans then the results can be subdivided into separate results chapters each focused on a particular specialist area; such as (1) construct development, (2) construct testing in pre-clinical models and (3) construct testing in the clinical setting, in the previous example. Splitting the results into chapters focuses the reader on the importance of the data shown in a particular chapter and is much easier for examiners to follow.

### Figure presentation

High quality figures complimented by clear and detailed legends, are essential to the persuasiveness of your results chapter. As a general rule, figures/legends should inform the reader of what your data is telling them without them having to refer to the written text sections of the results – the so called 'cover-up' test. Use professional artwork packages such as Adobe Illustrator to generate high quality images with a range of file export options. See Box 9.4 for guidance on making a good figure.

### Main text of your results

Results chapters have similarities to research papers in that each results chapter (should you decide to have more than one) is split into subsections. Each subsection should be titled with the main finding it will present. As always, present the data impartially and do not interpret it. Regarding figure

---

**Box 9.4** How to get a great figure

- All tables and axes to charts are clearly labelled.
- The magnification for images is documented (if appropriate) and the image is sharply in focus. Use arrows to indicate important features.
- Briefly introduce the method in the opening phrase.
- The correct statistical package/test has been used and clearly stated.
- Document the number of times an experiment was repeated, and detail whether the data uses pooled data from multiple experiments or is representative of one experiment over a set number performed.
- If animals or patients are used, ensure the cohort size is clearly mentioned.

---

placement – you have three options. You can either: insert figures throughout the text, insert figures at the end of the subsection text, or insert all figures at the end of the chapter. It's advisable to do either of the latter two, as this enables examiners to read without interruption and cross-check your writing and figures at the same time. As described earlier, theses with multiple results chapters often include short introductions and discussions after the results. This is your chance to introduce and contextualise the specific literature relevant to your chapter, and then draw out the implications of your findings in the focused discussion.

---

*Top tip*

Large file-size figures will slow or crash your word processer, avoid this by exporting your figures as compressed smaller files, for example, PNG format. Note, this may occasionally compromise image quality.

---

### Discussion

The discussion can be the most deceptive chapter when writing a thesis. One of the biggest pitfalls is reiteration of your results – this is not what a discussion should be. Discussions should embellish your results chapter highlighting the significance of your data in the context of your specialist field of research and the generic field more broadly. Most theses will contain several results chapters, each containing a focused discussion. Thus, the main discussion chapter can be quite concise at around 10 pages in length and should deliberate on how the data presented fits into your research field and questions at large. This is certainly the preference for most examiners. Alternatively, you may elect to have one large discussion chapter upwards of 20–30 pages.

Either way, pull out the key themes running through your thesis and embellish key background information that you touched on in your Introduction. It's important you show you've actually read key papers, not just sourced the abstracts online! Moreover, it's quite common for an examiner to ask for more detail on aspects of background information relevant to your experiments; this can be mitigated by comparing and contrasting the research approaches used in different studies to that of your own, and their potential impact on the results. The inclusion of diagrams (one or two) that summarise your key findings will help the reader better contextualise your results. For example, if you've discovered a new pathway that helps promote signalling through a cell molecule, draw a detailed diagram of current knowledge and where your data fits in. Diagrams aid both to break-up pages of text and consolidate information in a visually appealing manner.

### Conclusion/Future work

At the end of the main discussion, you should include a short summary or conclusion. This conclusion is a 'specialised' abstract, which ties all the results chapters together and highlights your main keynote finding(s). It should detail how the main findings enhance or transform understanding of the research field. This conclusion should not parrot the abstract, but does share similarities, most importantly keep it brief (300–400 words at most). Your thesis may include a future work section immediately after the conclusion. This should have 4–5 bullet points, with around a paragraph for each. These are relatively low value sections but as always, be sensible and concise. There's no point writing a great thesis and then coming up with shocking, implausible or bizarre future experiments; keep it straightforward and know when to stop talking – a critical transferable life skill.

### Selection of examiners

It's beyond the remit of this chapter to discuss the viva; however, while writing your thesis, inevitably your thoughts will wander as to who the internal and external examiners will be. Every supervisor is different in whether they will reveal their choice of examiners to the students prior to, during or after the write up of the thesis; and also how much input the student has into the decision. Thus, our comments here are based on our own personal perspectives:

*Allison*: As a supervisor, I am reluctant to tell my student who the internal and external examiner will be until the thesis is almost complete. The reason I delay providing this information is to prevent unconscious bias in the writing of the thesis; there is a risk that the student will focus their literature search around the examiners' research field at the expense of others. Once I am confident from viewing drafts that my students are giving a good unbiased account of the research field I tend to let them have a choice of five external examiners. From the list, I ask them if there is one examiner they know they would be uncomfortable with, and I exclude that person from my deliberations. Upon submission of the thesis, I reveal who the actual examiners will be. In this regard the student has a 'heads up' on potential examiners, and knows they had a say to a certain extent on the selection process. The defining point in my selection of examiners is my relationship with them; a strong relationship will enable me to judge their fitness to be an examiner: are they knowledgeable of the work my lab produces, respectful, fair and understanding of how challenging a PhD degree is. A viva should be a lively debate that, yes, challenges the student but does not leave them traumatised. I can honestly say that neither I, nor my students, have ever regretted my choice of examiners.

*Manu*: As a student, I experienced a similar relationship with my supervisor as Allison outlines. Though as my research field is rather small it was less difficult to imagine who could be my internal and external examiner. In addition, I agree that it is helpful that the examiners are scientists I know I could have a good scientific debate with, as opposed to an interrogation. One advantage can be the selection of an external examiner who you may have already met, for example at a conference or when they came to give a talk at your research institute. Someone you've had a conversation with, albeit brief, is less intimidating as an examiner than someone you only know from research papers. Nevertheless, over the years you will (hopefully!) have built a good rapport with your supervisor and must have faith in their judgement to select examiners that will enrich your viva.

## Conclusion

The final year of a PhD is the most important, you must be focused and aim to do two things: finish your experiments and start writing your thesis. Avoid getting side-tracked into new research areas by making a list of the remaining key experiments needed to strengthen your hypothesis and consolidate the data. Writing a thesis is challenging, requires discipline and at times can feel enormously tedious. But hang in there, once you create that PDF of your polished, professional thesis – the feeling of warranted pride will make it all worthwhile.

## Common pitfalls

1. *'I've run out of money and still have experiments left to do.'*
   During your final year of research, it's not uncommon to find yourself running out of resources including time and money. Your supervisor and/ or lab manager should be able to inform you of your consumables budget

and what funds you have remaining. This is often the best guide as to what experiments you're able to commit to before finishing your work. If you've run out of student bursary or stipend, it might be possible for your supervisor or department to provide you with extra funding, but this is rare and entirely at their discretion.

2. *'My thesis is 50 or 500 pages long.'*

When it comes to writing a thesis, there is no 'correct' length. Depending on your data, this is going to vary substantially in format. Examiners will be open minded as to the exact length, but there are boundaries, so if your thesis is 50 pages long there is something wrong – you haven't written enough. Likewise, if you've just crossed the 500-page threshold, you've written too much. As a guide, 200–250 pages (double spaced) is a reasonable target. Typical introductions will be around 50 pages; methods and materials around 15–20 pages, and concise discussions around 10 pages. This leaves you with approximately 120 pages to fill with results, which if in three separate results chapters comes at 40 pages each. If you're well under, check you've enough data to talk about and pad out your Introduction and discussion; if well over 250 pages, you need to drastically cut down – either in-text, figures or both; have you saturated your research narrative with information overload or do you have too many stories happening at once?

3. *'I don't want my internal/external examiner.'*

Though uncommon, it's not unheard of for students to take a particular view on either or both of their examiners. As discussed, much of this relies on the faith you place in your supervisor's judgement. However, if you hold strong concerns and are ready to justify them, discuss this with your supervisor and if necessary graduate school. Ultimately, it's in everyone's interest for the decision to be reached by consensus rather than imposition!

## Further reading

1. Dunleavy, P. *Authoring a PhD: How to Plan, Draft, Write and Finish a Doctoral Thesis or Dissertation.* Palgrave-Macmillan, 2003.
2. Murray, R. *How to Write a Thesis.* Open University Press, 2011.
3. Gustavii, B. *How to Prepare a Scientific Doctoral Dissertation based on Research Articles.* Cambridge University Press, 2012.

# Chapter 10 **The viva and moving on**

*Rachel Allen[1] and Kate Gowers[2]*

[1] Reader in Immunology of Infection and Head of Graduate School, St George's, University of London, UK

[2] Research Associate, University College London, UK

## Background

The viva examination should represent the final throes of your PhD, that last major hurdle before you escape to/embark upon your future career. Vivas can be enjoyable but are exhausting. In your viva, you should strive for a discussion of your work with two engaged examiners in which you showcase your findings and expertise. What you don't want is to find yourself tongue-tied or defensive in the face of bored or aggressive examiners. This chapter will help you prepare for the completion of your PhD and discuss future options to consider as you move on.

## An examiner's perspective (Rachel)

How does an examiner approach a PhD thesis? As soon as that large, padded envelop arrives I'll open it to check the accompanying paperwork for any pre-viva tasks, but the thesis itself will probably languish on my desk for several weeks. In spare moments, I might take a brief glance at the contents pages out of curiosity. I'll sit down to read a thesis 'properly' over a 2–3-day period within the week before the viva, so that I can appreciate it as a whole story with the contents fresh in my mind for the exam. First off, I'll read the Acknowledgements for a bit of light entertainment then on to the abstract followed by a check of the Table of Contents so I have a rough idea of the narrative to expect. Before getting properly stuck in, I'll count the number of pages in the Introduction chapter in order to time my first coffee break,

*How to Complete a PhD in the Medical and Clinical Sciences*,
First Edition. Edited by Ashton Barnett-Vanes and Rachel Allen.
© 2018 John Wiley & Sons Ltd. Published 2018 by John Wiley & Sons Ltd.

in the expectation that I'll be able to read that chapter in one sitting. Please note: 80+ pages of Introduction is likely to antagonise rather than inspire an examiner at this point.

I hope that the Introduction will give me a great insight into the theory and rationale that underpin your thesis, rather than providing 50-odd pages of generic background for me to wade through without any indication of what your research questions are or why they are important. I don't want to have to guess the relevance of what I'm reading during this early stage of my assessment. Other possible irritations for me as I work through a thesis include prolific typos (everyone has a few, but multiple typos per page are downright annoying) or figures that cost me unnecessary time and effort to interpret due to the lack of an appropriate figure legend. These distract my attention from the research itself, drag out the reading process and are unlikely to induce a friendly examiner state of mind.

A first read through will give me the general feel and meaning of a thesis, and possibly initiate a list of corrections to address any of the issues described here. The second and third read-throughs are when I evaluate the experimental approach in detail. What studies were performed and why? Do they address the research questions? How might things have been done differently? Have the results been interpreted appropriately? Are the conclusions justified? From these later read-throughs, I'll draw up a list of questions that I'd like to cover in the viva. Finally, on the day before/day of the viva I'll read through my notes again and scan through key parts of the thesis.

Immediately before the viva, the examiners discuss our individual opinions on the thesis, whether we think it's appropriate for the degree, which aspects need to be discussed and who will ask questions on which areas. Although we'll have agreed an approach, the nature of the questioning is also determined by the interactions between the candidate and the examiners. How you as a candidate respond to questions will influence your examiners' approach for subsequent questions; this will become more fluid as everyone becomes settled in the discussion. For example, we may switch between 'big picture' and detail-specific questions depending on your ability to answer (whether due to knowledge or nerves).

Examining a PhD takes up a large chunk of time and energy; reading the thesis, travelling to the exam, then listening to you talk about your work for a couple of hours or more before hauling back again to write a report. Given the time they have committed to this process, most examiners do want to have a pleasant experience, learn something interesting and enjoy a proper discussion about research. Bear this in mind for the viva – we'd much rather be energised by an in-depth conversation with an enthusiastic researcher than waste hours throwing questions at a monosyllabic one in an atmosphere of mutual resentment. Similarly, trawling through corrections is not a pleasant task for an examiner – we'll only ask for these if we think they're absolutely necessary.

## The viva

### Preparation

If you have followed the advice of Chapter 9, you won't have skewed your thesis towards over-referencing your examiners. But once your thesis has been submitted it is worth taking time to look over their work. This doesn't mean that you should memorise every paper they've written, but a scan of their publications can give you some idea of their interests or expertise and from that an indication of which particular aspects of your thesis they might hold most interest in. Read and re-read your thesis in order to familiarise yourself with everything in it and any statistical tests you have used. Try to look at your results critically: why did you use a particular technique instead of another one? What could you have done differently and what are the limitations of your data? You're almost certain to find typos at this point but don't worry, that's normal. Do keep a list of these, as you're likely to find some mistakes that have escaped your examiners' attention.

Revise key references, particularly ones that set the context at the outset of your project and those outlining any essential techniques you have used. Take particular care when reading through your Introduction, as this should be covered in the early stages of the exam. One common mistake is to include statements of fact or background that you don't fully understand, so make sure you're able to answer questions about or justify what you've written. You should also perform a literature search in the weeks before your viva to check for any important articles relevant to your work that may have been published since you submitted. Be aware of any contradictions between your work and published studies. Rehearse a 3–4-minute summary of your work – What were the research questions?; Why are they important?; What did you find?; Were there any surprise findings?; How is it all relevant? This will provide you with a useful summary of your work for the start of the viva. Try to arrange a practice viva, ideally with someone outside your supervisor team who can look at the work with fresh eyes and without bias. Practice vivas are often a grim experience, but you'll be more prepared for the real thing if you've done one.

### On the day

Know what to wear (see Box 10.1). Allow yourself plenty of time to find the room, speak to your supervisor and calm yourself down if necessary. Don't feel obliged to meet up with other lab members before the viva, as this can be an unnecessary distraction (often involving mythical viva horror stories) – you

**Box 10.1** What to wear/bring on the day of your viva

1. Wear professional attire (e.g. a suit)
2. Have a copy of your thesis (annotated)
3. Notepad and pens/pencils – so you can take notes of comments/ corrections
4. Water, as you might be talking for a couple of hours without a break.

can ask your supervisor to book a room that's off the beaten path in order to avoid this possibility.

## What to expect

Examiners are often asked to submit preliminary reports ahead of the viva to ensure that they have formed their own independent opinion of the work. Regardless, they will spend at least 15–20 minutes conferring with one another before asking you to join them. If you're lucky, they'll schedule this discussion before the official viva start time, but you will probably find yourself waiting around for a few minutes at least.

To ensure consistency and fairness, many universities have adopted the use of independent chairs and/or recording of PhD vivas. The purpose of an independent chair is to ensure that the viva is conducted appropriately rather than to ask questions or decide the outcome of the viva. In some institutions, it's also possible for your supervisor to attend, but this should be subject to your agreement. Check your university's exam regulations well in advance so that you know what to expect. Examiners can vary in approach depending on the number of times they have examined a thesis. More experienced examiners may have a tendency towards broad questions that allow them to consider how you place your work in the context of current knowledge. In contrast, inexperienced examiners have a reputation for nit-picking fine details and may have only their own thesis as a point of comparison (with or without a rose-tinted view of how good it was).

Most vivas will start gently with an opening question or two, designed to put you at ease, for example, why did you choose the project, did any particular findings surprise you and a request to give a brief overview of your work. This is the time to apply the 'elevator pitch' summary of your project, so don't go into excessive detail – that's what the rest of the viva is for and you don't want to lose their attention at the start. In addition to helping you settle into the viva, the examiners will also use these opening statements to assess how well you understand your project and its relevance. Depending on your examiner's experience and interests, they may continue with questions about some of your findings or experimental approaches in this initial discussion.

Don't be thrown by any tangential questions, there may not be a 'correct' answer but rather an opportunity to open a two-way discussion with your examiners in which you can demonstrate how you think as a researcher.

When they move on to the thesis, most examiners start with the Introduction followed by each chapter in turn but you can find yourself jumping back and forwards between chapters, particularly if directing the examiners to another part of the thesis helps you answer a question. Be prepared to talk through your experimental approach and analyses in detail as this is the means by which examiners will determine that the work you have presented is indeed your own. Your examiners may not agree with all the experimental approaches you used. If so, you should defend your work without being defensive. Give due consideration to any problems they highlight, but justify the reasons why you chose to adopt a particular approach and what advantages you think it may have had. Responses to avoid include: 'because my supervisor told me to' (unless you yourself can demonstrate that you understand the shortcomings); 'someone else did that and I don't understand why they did it that way'; or being defeatist – conceding every point without justification or discussion can give the impression that you don't understand your own work.

Be aware of verbal and non-verbal cues throughout the viva – if the examiners make repeated reassuring statements, it's possible that you're coming across as too negative or defensive. If necessary, modify the length of your answers. Be more concise if their eye contact drifts off during long answers. Lengthen your responses or ask whether more detail is required if each of your answers is met by a lengthy pause. Some universities set a maximum time limit for a PhD viva. You should expect something in the range of 2–3 hours, but a long viva is not necessarily a bad thing, it may just mean an enthusiastic discussion of an excellent thesis. At the end of the viva, you can expect your examiners to ask you to leave the room for a few minutes. They'll use this time to finalise their decision and debate the list of any corrections that will be required. One final point here – it's normal to feel exhausted and somewhat deflated after your viva, even if you've sailed through it. After all, you'll have spent a couple of hours in intense concentration, dealing with criticism of the project that you've committed several years of your life to. See Box 10.2 for a summary of top tips.

## Corrections

Most people will have to make some corrections to their PhD, even if only a few typos. Your examiners should provide you with a list of corrections immediately after the viva, or within a short time frame after that. However

---

**Box 10.2** Key tips for a viva

1. If you're not sure what they're asking, repeat and clarify the question.
2. Maintain a positive attitude and sufficient energy in your responses.
3. Remember that the point of a viva is to challenge you; don't become too defensive – difficult questions do not necessarily mean that the examiners disagree with your results or conclusions.
4. Treat it as a conversation rather than an interrogation (you can even ask your examiners questions about their opinions).
5. Don't pretend if you don't know the answer to a question, it is best to say so and to say what you do know about the subject – bluffing your way through a question will be apparent to the examiners and may irritate them.
6. Enjoy it if you can – this is probably the last time you'll have two expert researchers giving their full attention to your work in discussion.

---

exhausted you feel, try to clarify with the examiners what the corrections are (or are likely to be) immediately after the viva to make sure that you understand what they are looking for and whether both or only one of your examiners will need to approve them. Unless you have nothing more than a list of typos to correct, arrange a discussion with your supervisor to get their input and thoughts on how to approach your corrections. And most importantly, check whether there is a specified time limit in which you are required to submit them. You are encouraged to address these as a priority.

**Minor**

Minor corrections can range from sorting out a handful of typos to providing additional text, amending figures or a long list containing all the previous. You're likely to be expected to submit these corrections within 3 months or so of the viva and your examiners should believe that the work is 'minor' enough to be achievable within that time frame.

**Major**

Examples of major corrections include restructuring of a thesis, further background reading or a major re-analysis of results. If your examiners request major corrections, this is likely to involve a longer time frame, for example, up to 18 months and may or may not require a further viva examination. The decision regarding a further viva can be made once the examiners have read a resubmitted thesis. If you can, it's worth asking your supervisor to discuss the expected corrections with the examiners after the viva, as your energy and concentration may be lagging after the exam. Then arrange a follow-up meeting with your supervisors as soon as possible

**Box 10.3** Common corrections pitfalls

1. Failing to clarify the nature of the corrections that are expected.
2. Leaving corrections until just before the deadline.
3. Failing to consult with your supervisors before making and/or submitting corrections.

after the viva, so you can get their opinion and support for making the necessary corrections. Bear in mind that they retain their supervisory responsibility (and that you are entitled to university support) throughout the writing up and corrections process, until the completion of your degree studies. If you are not receiving suitable supervision through a corrections period, then contact your graduate school staff for advice. See Box 10.3 for common pitfalls.

**Fail**

A 'fail' outcome is extremely rare, but not impossible and might come with a recommendation that your work is considered for an MPhil degree. Your university should inform you whether you are allowed a further attempt to submit your thesis for a PhD, but contact administrators and graduate school staff for advice as early as possible. You can also check your degree regulations if you think that you have grounds for appeal, bearing in mind that there may be a time limit within which you can do this. Consider an appeal if there is evidence that the examination was not conducted appropriately or fairly; however, they are not an opportunity to challenge an examiner's academic judgement.

**Career routes**

You'll have had some thoughts on your long-term career at the time you applied for a PhD, but these may well have changed over the course of your studies. At least a year before you are due to complete your PhD, you should start making firm plans. By this point in time you should have some insight into your experience of academic research, the skills you have developed and what you might (or indeed might not) want to do next.

Whatever route you choose, planning ahead will allow you to fill in any gaps on your CV, visit laboratories and submit any necessary funding applications. If you want to move into a new area, seek out people who are working in that career for information and advice. One way to find these people is through the network of contacts you've established during your PhD – if you ask around among fellow students, post-docs and PIs in

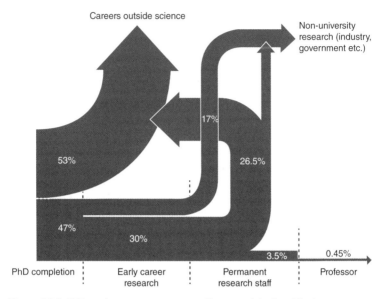

**Figure 10.1** PhD graduate career outcomes. Courtesy of the Royal Society

your institution someone is likely to know someone (who knows someone…) who has made a move in that direction and can put you in touch. Another route that can enable informal contact is through social media, but if you use this route make sure that your own profiles are professional or locked down… Finally, a range of 'career conferences for PhD graduates' exist, often attended by the great and the good of management consultancy and investment banking, these events can give you insight and connections in different industries. See Figure 10.1 for an analysis of PhD graduate outcomes in the UK.

## Academia

There's a lot more to academia than research, and a PhD can also equip you for various non-academic careers within the Higher Education sector. For example, your research background could be valuable for intellectual property, grant writing or grant management roles. Unless you're a research superstar cushioned by significant grant funding, an academic career will also involve a significant amount of teaching and/or administrative duties. You can put yourself ahead of the competition by starting to acquire experience in teaching and supervision, public engagement or committee service during your PhD. If you have been responsible for university teaching during your PhD, explore the possibility of gaining some form of accreditation for this, for example, Associate Fellowship of the Higher Education Academy. Your university may have frameworks in place to facilitate this.

The traditional scientific academic career route following a PhD is designed to progress through post-doc and/or fellowship positions before acquiring a highly competitive university job. By the final stages of your PhD you'll no doubt be aware of the high attrition rate along this path and you should also consider the impact that the necessary transitions in roles and perhaps locations may have on your personal life. A track record of publications and funding are of prime importance, so start early by applying for travel grants and fellowships during your PhD.

### Research-related careers: Industry

If you're keen to escape academia but wish to remain in the world of research, there are various options. These days, going 'into industry' often means working in a start-up rather than a traditional Big Pharma job. Start-up companies often arise from academic research, and so tend to be clustered in science parks near universities. The network of contacts acquired during your PhD may therefore help you in identifying and finding these kinds of jobs. In this environment, you can benefit from experience of corporate culture and utilise your technical skills, albeit directed more towards development than research.

### Research-related careers: Publishing

Science publishing is essential to the progress of science and can therefore be another alternative route of employment if you want to continue to be involved in scientific research with scientists, but you no longer want to be in the lab. Reading and contributing to scientific publications are big parts of doing a PhD so pursuing a career in publishing is often appealing to those considering careers outside the lab. Science publishing is a diverse industry and the jobs can be quite different depending on the organisation. It is worth taking some time to really understand what the different roles involve and what you'd be most suited to – whether it be as an editor of a research journal, selecting and reviewing manuscripts; or as an editor of a review journal, commissioning articles on cutting edge topics and helping the authors to construct their articles.

It is important to realise that editorial work is much less specialised than anything you will have done as a PhD student and takes place in the background; in contrast to the work you might have done leading the writing and publishing of articles during your PhD. However, having the opportunity to work with scientists who have a range of expertise, and to review and select manuscripts on a broad range of topics can be a rewarding and attractive alternative career path to scientific research. Editorial jobs usually require a PhD and at least some post-doctoral experience. During this time, get as much experience of science communication beyond the publication of research articles as you can. This could include writing blogs, writing science articles for magazines/university newspapers, peer reviewing papers, appraising manuscripts on appropriate websites or social media, editing other scientists' manuscripts before submission or working for companies who employ scientists to edit papers written by scientists for whom English is not their first language. It is important to show that you actively want to pursue a career in science publishing and that it is not just a fall back option. Should you decide to return to lab based science in the future, a period of time in the publishing industry will be highly valuable in informing your future manuscripts and publications.

### Non-scientific careers

While it's not possible to provide an exhaustive list of potential careers that are open to you if you decide that you want to move away from research, there are some more common ones that can make good use of the expertise gained during your PhD. Specialised areas of professions such as law (and particularly patent law), government policy, funding bodies, think-tanks and charity work, consultancy, PR and finance take advantage of PhD trained employees. If you're moving further afield, take some time to assess the wider set of skills you've acquired during your degree and how these might be relevant to your chosen career. These include problem solving, project management, communication skills and assimilating complex information. Identifying and evaluating your transferrable skills will help you in preparation for job applications and enable you to define what you can bring to a given role.

### Further study

Upon completion of a PhD, it's easy to assume that you'll never have (and at this point may never want) to study again. But depending on your career choice, it may be unavoidable. Success in your future career may require you to engage with Continuing Professional Development/Continuing Personal and Professional Development/Workforce Development or whatever your employer chooses to call it at the time. Indeed, academic careers increasingly require a formal teaching qualification or accreditation.

### Returning to clinical training

Depending on your PhD contract, you may have already been performing clinical duties or rotas on nights or weekends. However, if you've had the opportunity to forgo these commitments for a sustained period of time, getting back into the rhythm of clinical work may require a bit more effort. In the first instance, be clear on when your duties resume and what time in the week you will be able to dedicate to any outstanding PhD commitments. Clinicians are famed for a comparatively low rate of thesis write-ups and submissions – there is no point doing three or more years of work to not finish it at the end. If you've been unable to submit before returning to clinical practice, then dedicate your free time to doing so. Similarly, if you're undertaking an MB-PhD, your return to medical school is going to be a challenging readjustment. In the first instance, make sure your university is aware of your impending return, and that all enrolment and financial considerations/paperwork are in order. You may require a 'refresher' course, particularly if you're going back into ward work – most medical schools will be keen to provide you with this, or place you initially with a sympathetic clinical firm to restart your rotations. Again, if you've not submitted your thesis, you will have a difficult year writing up alongside clinical study – but you're not the first and won't be last, it can be done.

## Conclusion

Undertaking your viva is one of the most challenging components of your PhD. But you're unlikely to be in the room if you aren't ready, as your supervisor will have signed off on it. From this you should draw confidence. Be sure to take some rest after your viva, preferably once you've got your corrections in. From there on, it is down to you. A PhD is a gateway to jobs and careers in varied fields and countries, we wish you every success!

## Further reading

1. The Royal Society. 2010. The Scientific Century: securing our future prosperity. Available online at:https://royalsociety.org/topics-policy/publications/2010/scientific-century/(accessed 8 December, 2016).
2. Williams, K., Bethell, E., Lawton, J., Parfitt-Brown, C., Richardson, M., Victoria, R. *Completing your PhD – Pocket Study Skills*. Palgrave-Macmillan, 2010.
3. *The Guardian*. 2015. How to survive a PhD viva: 17 top tips. Available online at: https://www.theguardian.com/higher-education-network/2015/jan/08/how-to-survive-a-phd-viva-17-top-tips (accessed 8 December, 2016).
4. Vitae. 2016. Defending your doctoral thesis: the PhD viva. Available online at: https://www.vitae.ac.uk/doing-research/doing-a-doctorate/completing-your-doctorate/your-viva (accessed 8 December, 2016).

# Chapter 11   Phds in veterinary science and medicine

Fiona Cunningham[1], Jonathan Elliott[2],
Fiona Tomley[3] and Kristien Verheyen[4]

[1] Professor of Pharmacology, Royal Veterinary College, UK

[2] Professor of Veterinary Clinical Pharmacology and Vice Principal for Research and Innovation, Royal Veterinary College, UK

[3] Professor of Experimental Parasitology, Royal Veterinary College, UK

[4] Senior Lecturer in Clinical Epidemiology and Head of Graduate School, Royal Veterinary College, UK

## Background

Having chosen a PhD project in the field of veterinary science/medicine, you'll quickly come to realise just how broad a term this is. You and fellow PhD students will be addressing research questions that aim to advance current understanding of a diverse range of issues relating to the health and wellbeing of livestock, companion, zoo or wild animals. This may involve working at the cellular and molecular level, using whole (individual or groups of) animals of different species or breeds, or gathering and modelling data at the population level. Topics of interest include aspects of animal physiology such as structure and motion, welfare, genomics and genetics, pathogenesis, diagnosis and treatment of disease (including species or breed variability in disease susceptibility and response to therapeutic agents) and the epidemiology, surveillance and control of infectious diseases. Novel vaccine development and food security are also important issues in veterinary science/ medicine. Many PhDs in this field operate within the 'one health' context which recognises that the health and wellbeing of animals, humans and the ecosystem are interconnected. Therefore, the projects are often attractive to both veterinary graduates and those with Bachelor's or Master's degrees in a range of subjects including bioveterinary, biomedical or animal sciences, one health and epidemiology.

If you're studying full-time, the likelihood is that you'll be based at one of the eight veterinary schools in the UK, all but one of which are part of a larger

*How to Complete a PhD in the Medical and Clinical Sciences,*
First Edition. Edited by Ashton Barnett-Vanes and Rachel Allen.
© 2018 John Wiley & Sons Ltd. Published 2018 by John Wiley & Sons Ltd.

**Box 11.1** A student's view – external institution training

Being a PhD student based at another institution is a great opportunity to experience research in practice, outside of a university setting. However, being physically isolated from the university research group and other PhD students can be a little daunting, especially if you are unaware that other students may be having similar setbacks to those that you are experiencing. Making the effort to attend university run courses or finding alternatives at your institution requires good self-motivation to progress your PhD skillset, which is especially important in the first year of study. You get out of your PhD as much as you are willing to put in.

Danica Pollard

university. However, you could be located in, or spend the majority of your time at, an external research institute or centre that has links to, or is affiliated with, one of the schools (see Box 11.1). There are also animal charities and government organisations undertaking research into animal health and disease that host PhD students who are registered at one of the veterinary schools or universities. Wherever you find yourself, you're certain to be working alongside postgraduate students and researchers from a diversity of backgrounds and there should be plenty of opportunity to expand your knowledge of many areas of research in veterinary science/medicine beyond the topic you've selected for your PhD.

Despite the exciting times that lie ahead of you over the next 3–4 years (or the equivalent in part-time study), there will be challenges along the way. The purpose of this chapter is to cover key areas relevant to a veterinary science or medicine PhD student, complimenting guidance offered elsewhere in this book.

## Is it for me?

If you're a veterinary graduate, the hands-on experience of research you gained during your undergraduate degree programme may have been somewhat limited. This might mean quite a steep learning curve at the start of your PhD, particularly if your project is largely, or entirely, laboratory based (see Box 11.2). You may be working alongside science graduates who started their PhD at the same time as you and who have not only undertaken a final year project, but also one or more research placements out-with their course such as summer studentships. Some of your fellow PhD students may have done a year's research as part of an MSci or an MRes degree. Therefore, if you compare yourself with them at the outset, you may feel at a substantial disadvantage. However, do bear in mind that during your undergraduate studies and any time spent in clinical practice you will have acquired a range of

---

**Box 11.2** A student's view – bedding in

As a veterinary graduate starting a lab based PhD I was worried that my lack of experience would be a real disadvantage. Many skills that other students found easy, such as using a pipette, were new to me. However, after a few weeks in the lab I felt like I'd been doing it for years.

Alana Burrell

---

**Box 11.3** A student's view – defining your schedule

It is true that many vets will have developed time management skills in general practice but these are usually within a quite rigid framework – consultations for several hours, operations and dealing with hospitalised patients between certain times and so on. You are continually developing new skills but these are in response to problems presented to you in the form of difficult cases to treat or discuss with owners. With the PhD, there is often no framework for how you should spend your time and it is up to you to fill it and plan your days appropriately, which is quite different. Self-motivation and the ability to drive the research project forwards independently are therefore extremely important.

Jack Lawson

---

generic (professional) skills. Many of these skills such as time management, problem solving, prioritising tasks and summarising complex information in writing or verbally, are transferable to research and you will find them invaluable in helping you to successfully complete your PhD (see Box 11.3).

Something else to consider is that *any* PhD project or programme of study will almost certainly include one or more elements that the individual undertaking it will find time consuming, repetitive and/or tedious. This will happen regardless of their undergraduate degree training *but* if you're a veterinary medicine graduate, you may have decided to leave practice because you've become disenchanted with the routine nature of much of the work and with the long hours. If so, you could be a little disappointed with your PhD project initially should you find that although the nature of the work is quite different, these features are still evident. Some vets also miss the more rapid reward associated with 'finding and fixing' problems for animals and their owners daily. Therefore, being motivated to answer the underlying research question(s) posed in the doctoral project is essential. On the plus side, you may well find it very satisfying to be able to focus on one topic and study it in great depth, as this is likely to be rather different to your experience on the veterinary course and in practice. However, it can take a bit of adjusting to, so don't be tempted to take on too many 'side-projects', particularly in the first year of your PhD.

> **Box 11.4** A student's view – the rollercoaster
>
> Doing a PhD can be stressful and the work hours can be very long at times but this is offset by studying a subject you have a passion for. While I sometimes struggle with why something has gone wrong, when you do create new data or add to current understanding, there is a great sense of personal satisfaction.
>
> James Pritchard

## Your project

### Impact

All researchers like to believe that their contribution to the field they have chosen to investigate will have some meaningful impact; PhD students studying veterinary science/medicine are no different (see Box 11.4). Indeed, one of the reasons for selecting a particular project that's often given at interview is that the applicant can see the potential for the research outputs to make a difference. For some, the impact may be significant, potentially immediate, and can be on a national or international scale. Examples include bringing about a change in prescribing practice or in a method of disease control. However, the impact of the work will often be more modest and/or less immediate, for example when the PhD project is investigating molecular or cellular aspects of disease pathogenesis, or a potential new drug/vaccine target. Although it can be a little disheartening to study alongside someone whose work is receiving a lot of external interest, it certainly doesn't mean another PhD project is any less worthwhile. You may be one of the many PhD students working in the field of veterinary science/medicine who's being funded by the institution they are registered with, or an external funding body. This means your project will have been scrutinised by a review committee prior to the funding being awarded, and who have therefore been persuaded of the value of the work. Similarly, for self-funded projects, such as those that may be proposed by a vet who wishes to study on a part-time basis while remaining in practice, the institution where they are registered and their supervisors will have seen and approved the proposed aim of the research, the objectives and the approaches to be taken.

### Knowledge base

Your PhD project may have emerged, or evolved, from your supervisor's ongoing research. Alternatively, it may address a gap in existing knowledge which could lead to new research avenues, perhaps in a different species or to a related disease in the same species. Regardless of the origin of the idea(s) for your project, there will be some topics in veterinary science/medicine that are very well researched and others where limited information is available. In addition, papers that describe findings in laboratory animals or human, which are generally in far greater abundance, may prove to be irrelevant or even misleading. Moreover, there are many and varied species and breed differences at all levels from the sub-cellular (e.g. the profile of CYP isoenzymes in the liver responsible for metabolising drugs and toxins) through to the whole animal (e.g. in how different animal species move, or in the behavioural responses of groups of animals). If you're working on an under-researched topic or using certain domestic animal species (e.g. horses and donkeys) or wild animals, you could potentially produce data that breaks new ground. However, you may well have had to spend far more time establishing simple – but nevertheless very valuable – baseline data. In addition, while such data might be entirely novel in relation to that veterinary issue, species or breed, it can be perceived by some researchers as not being at the cutting edge.

## Reagents

It can be frustrating working with samples (e.g. blood, cells or tissues) from certain species if they are not commonly used by the majority of researchers in a field for whom the primary species of interest is human. You can come across unexpected and on occasions apparently inexplicable differences, such as a widely used technique that simply doesn't work. Another potential problem can be the lack of commercially available species-specific reagents such as antibodies and peptides/proteins or detection kits (e.g. ELISAs). This may mean that you have to spend much more time optimising a method or validating an assay before you can use it; or finding a company that will synthesise a protein/peptide of interest; or even having to do so yourself. Don't be disheartened by this. From the research training perspective, the experience of having to optimise a set of conditions is a valuable one. Moreover, if you've carried out the experiments properly using appropriate controls, the developmental approach you've taken can be included in your thesis. Something else to remember is that knowing a particular reagent, compound or approach either *doesn't* work at all, or not particularly well, can be helpful to others – so it is important to communicate your results, even when they are negative.

## Animal genomes

Genomic studies in animals are widespread and although the primary purpose will vary, an underlying aim is often to understand the biological function(s) of one or more of the genes in a genome, the proteins they encode and the underlying molecular mechanisms. While the genomes of a number of important domestic species have been sequenced, the extent to which they have been annotated varies, and the annotation is far less advanced than that of the human or mouse genomes. Your project may benefit from the use of one of the powerful research tools now available for genomic studies (see Chapter 4). However, they are expensive so if the cost of purchase and use has not been included in the original PhD proposal, the funding required may either not be available or may take a lot of time and effort to secure (see next section).

## Funding

In general, there's less funding available from charitable sources or industry for veterinary research than for studying problems relating to human medicine; this can make sourcing additional funds for consumables, equipment or travel to conferences more problematic. That said, pharmaceutical companies that manufacture and supply veterinary medicinal products, foodstuffs for livestock and horses or diets for (primarily) small animals, *are* interested in supporting veterinary research. Indeed, your PhD may have an industrial partner and there will be an opportunity to spend at least 3 months with the company. Examples of this include the iCASE (collaborative awards in science and engineering) and the industrial case partnership award scheme funded by the BBSRC (Biotechnology and Biological Sciences Research Council). If you hold one of these competitively awarded studentships, do make the most of the opportunities to interact with the industrial partner. Whether the company is a large multinational or a small/medium size enterprise, you will gain valuable insights into how research in industry is performed and what the drivers are.

If you're presenting your work at a conference and hoping to obtain some additional external funding for the trip, the range of options available to you should be the same as for any PhD student. Thus, with your supervisor's agreement, you could consider approaching the conference organisers, a learned society that you belong to as a student member or the organisation sponsoring your PhD studentship and/or the project. If it's an applied project that's not industrially sponsored, a company may well be prepared to sponsor your attendance; note that they will expect such support to be acknowledged on your poster or slides.

## Presenting and publishing your findings

Supervisors are keen for their PhD students to present their data at conferences and to write up their findings for publication. Despite the possible stressors associated with presenting and with networking and socialising if you don't know many/any of the other participants, attending a meeting is usually a great experience.

Chapter 8 covers presenting and publishing as a PhD student in detail. However, there is one situation not addressed there that, as someone working in the field of veterinary science/medicine, you may experience. That is when having submitted a piece of work that appears to be a good 'fit' with the conference theme, you find that it's very clearly not of mainstream interest. For example, you could be presenting an interesting and novel finding in horses with respiratory dysfunction at an international meeting attracting thousands of researchers and clinicians working on lung disease. You learn a great deal from the other presentations *but* the vast majority of participants are interested in human diseases, and even those who use animal models may show very limited interest in your work simply because it's in horses. Don't be put off by this. You may have to try that bit harder to engage others in what you have to say in your talk or on your poster but it will almost certainly be worth the effort, particularly if the feedback you receive provides you or listeners with an alternative view and fresh ideas for future studies or collaborations.

## Post-PhD, what's next for me?

If you're a veterinary graduate with an interest in research, deciding when to do your PhD might not have been a straightforward decision. You may have been aware of a few veterinary (or medical) students intercalating a PhD during their undergraduate degree, or going straight on to do a PhD after completing the course without spending any time in practice. More commonly though, veterinary graduates return to study on a full-time basis after having spent a bit of time in practice; those who've been in practice for longer may choose to study part-time or to undertake a professional doctorate in veterinary practice.

If you're a veterinary graduate who's opted to spend 3–4 years in full-time study, you may be doing a PhD with a view to returning to clinical practice and undertaking clinical research armed with a greater depth of understanding about your chosen topic and research methodology. Alternatively, you may be considering a career as a clinical lecturer in one of the veterinary schools. If this is the career path you intend to follow, and you haven't already undertaken specialist clinical training, your next step is likely to be an internship and/or a residency programme. If so, and you see it being a significant component of your future career, then look for one that offers the opportunity to engage in some research. Doing so will allow you to build on the research skills you've gained during your PhD, continue to publish and to develop useful collaborations. In addition, spending a period of time as a post-doctoral scientist before applying for specialist clinical training and/or a lectureship will aid your future development as an independent researcher. That said, there are plenty of other options (see Table 11.1) you can pursue once you've obtained your degree, and many different ways in which the research skills training you've received over the course of your PhD can be put to good effect. A similar range of options are available to PhD students who've come from a background in the bioveterinary, biomedical or animal sciences (see Table 11.1). As a science graduate with a veterinary science/medicine PhD, you'll be in a position to think about applying for a

**Table 11.1** Examples of post-PhD career paths

| First Degree | PhD Topic (area of veterinary science/ medicine) | Careers |
|---|---|---|
| Veterinary medicine | Basic or applied studies of a veterinary issue, particularly disease diagnosis/pathology/ patho-physiology or treatment | Clinical or pathology lectureship (specialist clinical training an advantage/a requirement if the role involves clinical service work) |
| Veterinary medicine | Veterinary epidemiology/public health | Animal disease surveillance/ policy work in a government/ non-government organisation; Non-clinical lectureship |
| Veterinary medicine | Basic or applied studies of any veterinary issue | First opinion or referral practice; Clinical work with an animal charity |
| Veterinary medicine *or* biomedical, bioveterinary or animal science | Basic or applied studies of any veterinary issue | Lectureship in a para-clinical or basic sciences discipline (post-doctoral study essential unless it is a teaching-only position) |
| Veterinary medicine or biomedical, bioveterinary or animal science | Basic or applied studies of any veterinary issue | Post-doctoral research position in academia, research institution, government organisation or registered charity |
| Veterinary medicine or biomedical, bioveterinary or animal science | Basic or applied studies of any veterinary issue | Industry (human or animal health): Research; Product management; Clinical trials |
| Veterinary medicine or biomedical, bioveterinary or animal science | Basic or applied studies of any veterinary issue | Scientific communication; Scientific events management; Public engagement etc. |
| Veterinary medicine or biomedical, bioveterinary or animal science | Basic or applied studies of any veterinary issue | Publishing (e.g. science writer; editorial role) |
| Veterinary medicine or biomedical, bioveterinary or animal science | Basic or applied studies of any veterinary issue | Research management (e.g. grants officer); Research administration (to include postgraduate student training) |

non-clinical lectureship in a veterinary school or other Higher Education institution. However, if the post you're interested in involves research and teaching, in order to be competitive, you will almost certainly need to have held one or two post-doctoral positions. These may be in the same or a different field to that which you studied during your PhD, but you will need to be investigating a topic that's likely to attract external funding. It can also be a good idea to carry out your post-doctoral research in a different group or institution from that in which you studied for your PhD; to others, this signals the start of your development as an independent researcher. A period spent working in another country can also help to broaden your experience of different research environments (see Chapter 12).

Whether you're a veterinary or a non-veterinary graduate, you may have thoroughly enjoyed doing your PhD in veterinary science/medicine but after having obtained your degree, feel ready for a change in direction. This could involve choosing a different topic to research at post-doctoral level, for example in the field of human health. Indeed, you may be faced with little choice if you're unable to secure long-term external funding to continue your research in veterinary science/medicine. Alternatively, you may consider leaving research altogether to work in a field where the transferable skills you've gained during your PhD studies can be put to good use. Therefore, do ensure that you make the most of the transferable skills training available to you as part of your PhD programme. Some examples of career options are given in Table 11.1 but there are many more possibilities. To quote Steve Hutchinson, PhD 'A doctorate equips you to pretty much have a go at anything – as long as you can sell the skill set that you have'[1].

## Conclusion

Undertaking a PhD in veterinary science or medicine can be an enjoyable and unique experience among the wider medical sciences. Your opportunity to work on diverse issues concerning a range of large animals and species will bring you into contact with myriad departments, researchers and agencies. However, the challenge of securing funding, coupled with the difficulty engaging in a wider medical science environment that is focused on human disease, necessitates your full commitment to the project and field.

## Possible concerns

1. *Maintaining your clinical skills*
   If you're a veterinary graduate, you may be a little worried that the calibre of your clinical skills will diminish over the 3–4 years of a full-time PhD, especially if it involves very little or no work with patients. Taking on a

limited amount of locum work might be an option for you because through doing so, you ought to be able to maintain a core level of technical skills although, of course, this will be an additional call on your time. Should you find that what you are able to do isn't sufficient, changing to part-time study *may* be an option. However, this would require the agreement of your supervisor(s) and of any external funder(s). There may be a very good reason(s) why such a move isn't possible so you shouldn't make the assumption that it will be an option when starting your PhD.

2. *Doing a PhD in veterinary science as a science graduate*
   If you're a science graduate who's working on a project that has a significant clinical focus, you may find that getting to grips with the background literature describing the pathophysiology and presentation of the disease state you're studying a little daunting at first. Moreover, if your main supervisor is a practising clinician, you might feel that s/he expects you to be as familiar with this as a veterinary graduate would have been. Don't worry too much. All PhD students should expect to read around the subject, particularly in the first year. Your supervisor will be able to direct you to appropriate literature and there are bound to be other people whom you can ask to explain any aspects that you're unclear about.

3. *Meeting with your supervisor*
   You might find that your clinical supervisor won't be as readily accessible to provide advice as one who doesn't have clinical duties. It may mean them not being available on certain days of the week throughout the year or for blocks of time. Therefore, it's essential that you agree a time of day/ day of the week and method of contacting them, and have also identified an alternative source of advice. This may be a post-doctoral scientist in the group (who might even have been asked to help supervise your project) but clinical projects can be co-supervised by a clinician-researcher who is laboratory based, or a basic scientist, who will fulfil this role. Either way, it is essential that you receive regular supervision; if you are not, speak to your graduate school.

## Acknowledgements

We thank Alana Burrell, Jack Lawson, Danica Pollard and James Pritchard. for their valuable contributions to this chapter and Sarah Allen for reading and commenting on the text.

## Reference

1. Vitae. Researcher career stories: Steve Hutchinson. Available online at: https://www.vitae.ac.uk/researcher-careers/researcher-career-stories/steve-hutchinson (accessed 8 December, 2016).

# Chapter 12 International perspectives on medical and clinical science PhDs

*Célia A. Soares[1] and Paul Langford[2]*

[1] MD-PhD Candidate, School of Health Sciences, University of Minho, Portugal

[2] Professor of Paediatric Infectious Diseases, Imperial College London, UK

## Background

There are many motivations for undertaking a PhD (or part of it) abroad. These can be a mix of the professional (networks, papers, presentations) and personal (beaches, caipirinhas and so on). As tempting as all these sound, going abroad for part or all of your PhD requires serious consideration. You'll need to adapt to new cultures or languages, and endure the isolation (or relief) of being away from family and friends for extended periods of time.

The two broad scenarios for you to navigate will be either completing the whole PhD internationally ('Full-PhD'); or just part of it (sometimes described as 'Dual-PhDs'). In this chapter, we'll cover these together and point out specific caveats for those undertaking each route. While PhD projects can be very challenging, undertaking them on home soil offers a stability and support network often vital to a student's success. In an international project, this won't be immediately available and places even greater importance on the decision you make – this chapter is here to help inform that process. Finally, alongside academic considerations (and general fun), a period of research overseas can serve as a time for immense personal growth, a point we touch on at the end of this chapter.

## Choosing a country

Unsurprisingly, deciding which country to go to is by far the most important decision you'll make regarding an international PhD; 'Anywhere but here' won't cut it. The following are important to factor into your decision.

---

*How to Complete a PhD in the Medical and Clinical Sciences,*
First Edition. Edited by Ashton Barnett-Vanes and Rachel Allen.
© 2018 John Wiley & Sons Ltd. Published 2018 by John Wiley & Sons Ltd.

## Duration and content

The duration of a PhD differs between countries. In Asia and Europe, they typically last 2–4 years. In contrast, in the USA a PhD student can take over 5 years to be awarded a doctorate. Further, expectations on PhD students can vary significantly. For example, in the US, students may perform techniques and projects that can take years to develop, compared to the sometimes shorter and more finite projects experienced in Europe. While all PhDs involve in-depth research, certain countries include a curriculum of classes often taken in the early years of a PhD, which may include preparatory work or assessments; further, in certain countries PhD students are expected to teach alongside research and class commitments.

## Language

Obvious as it is, pay attention to the location and language of the country you're considering: hand gestures work at a bar but won't get you far in the lab. Check whether the laboratory you're considering is internationally diverse and if so what language skills you might need. For example, if you are going to travel across Japan, speaking Japanese is a highly preferable. However, if you'll only be working in a Tokyo research unit, you might be able to get away with the basics if you have a good command of English. Needless to say, if you're conducting a clinical project you will need excellent command of the local language(s) (discussed later). While Europe and North America are the most popular destinations to look for a PhD, scientific opportunities are becoming increasingly widespread, including across Asia, Africa and Australasia; particularly with the increasing acceptance that 'tropical medicine should be done in the tropics'.

## Work ethos

Finally, it's worth considering the characteristics of the working culture in your new destination and how it might suit your aims and personality. For instance, some laboratories exert tight control over working hours and not everybody fits this *modus operandi*. Other projects might expect a minimum number of papers to be published in order for the PhD to be awarded – a pressure of expectation that doesn't work for everyone.

## Finding a department

Details on finding a supervisor and laboratory have been covered in Chapter 2 – here we will discuss issues specifically relating to going abroad.

Making the odd trip to New York, Singapore or Abuja is more difficult and expensive to come by than say, an underground tube to East London.

Thus, where possible, take any opportunity going to scope out in advance the institutions you're considering applying to. You might have a chance as an undergraduate or Master's student to take optional projects and rotations abroad or to participate in an official summer research programme. Table 12.1 highlights several examples of summer research internships. Either way, these are invaluable for gaining first-hand insight into your possible destination, as well as face time with your would-be supervisors and colleagues.

Official research programmes often guarantee you a small project with mentorship, funding and the opportunity to interact with students. You may be required to deliver a report or presentation at the end, which you should use as an opportunity to impress your potential future hosts. If no official programme exists, contact the lab of interest directly or through your home institution and offer your services for the summer. By showing initiative you might already be demonstrating your future suitability.

Once you've figured out where you want to go, the next step is getting there. If you don't already have good connections with the institution you wish to attend, contact members of your faculty or current mentors, explain your plan and map out their networks and which contacts they could introduce you to. LinkedIn or Research Gate could be helpful in this process. Alongside online networking, building up face to face connections can be immeasurably helpful – attend conferences and talk to researchers. Even if their field of work is not yours, they might be able to connect you to someone in a field more closely related. Remember to build connections with junior as well senior researchers; while senior researchers will make the decisions, junior researchers in departments might be more receptive to your questions and could offer invaluable signposting and advice.

## 'Full' PhDs versus 'dual-PhDs'

### Full PhD

Here, your scientific training is performed at a single institution. Prospective students can apply either to an institutional PhD programme or directly to a PhD position. In PhD programmes, students are selected to perform their research training, often through attending classes and rotating among different laboratories. After building your experience, you'll 'match' with a lab to conduct research towards a PhD thesis. In this scenario, the focus of your PhD may not be decided from the outset. For example, in the UK this may take the form of a '1 + 3' format, which includes a Master's year of rotations followed by 3 years of PhD research. Students applying directly to a PhD position will be presenting themselves as an 'off-the-shelf' researcher.

**Table 12.1** International summer internships for undergraduate science students

| Programme | Applicants | Host Institutions | Duration | Expenses |
|---|---|---|---|---|
| Welcome Trust – Biomedical Vacation Scholarship | Undergraduates from a university in UK or the Republic of Ireland | Supervisor in UK and Republic of Ireland, proposed by the student | 6–8 weeks | Stipend: £250 per week. Research expenses are not provided. |
| Amgen Scholars – US | Undergraduates – US citizens or US permanent residents | Selected institutions in US | ~8 weeks See local institution | All expenses covered. |
| Amgen Scholar – Europe | Undergraduates from European institutions participating in the Bologna Process | Selected institutions in Europe | ~8 weeks See local institutions | Coverage varies between institutions. |
| Amgen Scholars – Japan | Undergraduates worldwide | Selected institutions in Japan | ~8 weeks See local institution | Most of expenses covered. No health insurance coverage. |
| International Federation of Medical Students Association (IFMSA) – Research Exchange | IFMSA medical students worldwide | Selected IFMSA institutions worldwide | Minimum: 4 weeks See local institution | Students pay a fee to participate in the Exchange Programmes. Coverage varies between institutions. |

You won't have much say over the topic of your PhD, which is likely to be defined already by the lab and grant. In this scenario, you're likely to start swiftly on your PhD research.

## Dual PhD

By design, 'dual PhD' research is performed at two or more institutions in different countries. In theory, these schemes have been established to leverage the opportunities offered by international research while providing the necessary support for students, rather than them 'going it alone'. For departments and supervisors, these projects can serve both as a direct boost to their work, by providing you the chance to access techniques or equipment not readily available in one country; and also by serving to bring two institutions and their respective assets closer together for future larger collaborative projects. For you, the student, this type of PhD is typically supported by an administrative set up that coordinates the transition between the different periods and locations of research. For example, you may undertake training and classes at one institution and the PhD research at another, or be expected to split your time equally between the two institutions. It may involve multiple sites to attend and multiple co-supervisors. These schemes are not run across all institutions, but that doesn't mean you can't organise one with (a lot of) effort. Those who want some research experience abroad but aren't willing to commit to a full 3+ years should consider this option.

## Going abroad on a 'home' PhD

Finally, while a full- or dual-PhD abroad is a guaranteed method to gain international research experience; you can always do it yourself while studying at home. For example, aside from conferences, students take short trips to visit other institutions abroad to learn specific techniques or work on a particular research model. Bear in mind, you're more likely to have this opportunity if your supervisor(s) and lab have good international connections.

## Interviewing in a lab abroad

Interviews have been covered in detail in Chapter 2. Largely, the same rules apply: know your science background well and be able to explain both your motivation for wanting to take on a particular project and how your background is relevant to it. Further, be clear on the track record and ambitions of the department you wish to join. However, there are a few extra caveats to watch out for when applying for a PhD abroad:
• *Country knowledge*: Make sure you understand the recent history and geographical location of the country you wish to join. This should be near

impossible to not know if you've travelled for your interview; however, if it's taking place via Skype, make sure you know where it is on a map – *before* they ask.

- *Language skills*: We've all heard the classic story of a prospective French undergraduate being interviewed in German to throw them off. Though unlikely to happen in a science interview, make sure you're truthful in your application regarding your language abilities. It is likely they'll test them at interview, and frankly, 'Errrrrr' doesn't sound good in any language.
- *Non-academic interests*: Alongside your personality, science credentials and language skills, many interviewers will want to know what you do on a day off. Come prepared with some extracurricular activities and what motivates you to do them – if you don't have any, find some, quick! Be mindful that the value interviewers attach to outside interest varies, but for certain countries this can be significant.
- *Making good impressions*: It's common for prospective international students to meet different members of the lab or faculty members in the same department. In general, their opinions are highly valued and constitute a major factor in determining whether you'll be accepted in the team: so be nice. Often these lab members will take you on a tour of the facilities or present aspects of their project. You should ask valid questions about both.

## Funding

Most PhD Programmes or PhD positions already have secured funding for a student salary. But you may still need to apply for grants, perhaps to cover consumables or tuition fees. PhD fellowships may be awarded by government or private foundations; many have nationality restrictions. For example, the Fullbright Scholar Program accepts students from over 155 countries to perform their scientific training in US. Most dual-PhD programmes subsidise travel expenses, including to interview abroad. Alongside funding from foundations, pharmaceutical companies also offer travelling fellowships and other financial support. Table 12.2 includes typical costs PhD students may face in the US, UK and Germany. These figures are illustrative and may vary considerably.

## Administrative issues

### Status

For administrative purposes, there are multiple positions that can be attributed to visiting students: 'non-degree student', 'visiting scholar', 'officer', 'fellow' and so on. These titles can impact on your day-to-day issues, such as

**Table 12.2** Estimated costs of living in the US, UK and Germany as a PhD student in 2017

| Costs in US | |
| --- | --- |
| Travelling | $200–2500 |
| SEVIS Registration (US student database) | $200 once |
| Visa fees | $180–200 per application |
| University computer fees | $180/term |
| University registration fees | $150/term |
| Tuition fees | Covered by supervisor or Programme |
| Health insurance | ~$4000/year |
| Housing | $500–2000/month |
| Living expenses | $300–1000/month |
| **Costs in UK** | |
| Travelling | £50–1500 |
| Visa Fees (outside European Economic Area) | £322/application |
| University application fee | £50/once |
| Alumni society membership | £52/once |
| Tuition fees | £6000–26 000 |
| Housing | £400–2000/month |
| Living expenses | $300–1000/month |
| **Costs in Germany** | |
| Travelling | €50–1500 |
| Visa fees | €60 per application |
| Tuition fees | Public Institutions: Free |
| | Private Institutions: up to €30 000 |
| Semester Contribution (includes transportation, administrative fees and facilities fees) | €150–250/semester |
| Health insurance | 18% of salary or €60–160/month |
| Housing | €200–1000/month |
| Living expenses | €300–1000/month |

opening a bank account or the type of housing you can apply for. If you have an interest in taking classes, your position will determine whether you can attend. Some institutions offer visiting students the option of registering as an official student, paying tuition fees and taking classes for credits. Other institutions offer their employees, but not students or officers the opportunity to undertake classes for credit without the payment of fees. Another option is auditing (observing) classes without paying fees or getting credits. In some countries, PhD students have a job contract with the same rules as any other and therefore require paying health insurance, taxes and other contributions, negotiating days off and so on. Again, this is not the case everywhere so check well in advance on what your status will be – you don't want to be 'the student that slept in the lab' because your accommodation forms aren't sorted (there's always one…).

## Health care and assessments

The health care laws of a host country are complex and vary significantly, so take time to understand the rules and how they'll apply to you. Basic things to consider are whether you need to register for healthcare and if so where, what costs this might incur and the insurance options available to you. Your Office for International Affairs or equivalent (see below) or your supervisor can offer guidance. Many institutions have their own health insurance plans. Remember, this could depend on your institutional status. It is common practice for new lab staff to attend an occupational health appointment when joining a lab. You might need to show your medical records including vaccinations. Be aware that some countries have restrictions on the entry of international personnel with infectious diseases, and may request pre-arrival tests such as for HIV, methicillin-resistant *Streptococcus aureus* (MRSA) or vaccines like seasonal flu. It's essential you deal with these considerations in advance, the last thing you want after all this effort is being barred from entering the laboratory (or country!) pending health approval.

## The local office for international affairs

Most institutions have an Office of International Students/Affairs or the equivalent, and it's essential you get on first name terms with their staff as soon as possible. They'll deal with anything from visa paperwork, to flight advice and accommodation. In some institutions, they have a more formal role, for example, reminding you of key milestones to be met during your PhD. Check their websites for step-by-step guides and forums to interact with other international students. Look out for cultural activities for international students, including 'expat' events and offers or discounts to take advantage of.

## Maintaining clinical contact

PhD student schedules are busy but you may wish to maintain your clinical skills overseas. This could be simply keeping up to date with new medical guidelines or teaching clinical demonstrations and so on. Some trainees might want to dedicate some time during their PhD to maintaining hands on clinical training, but this must be planned carefully with your supervisor and department – note that there could be ethical or legal barriers to achieving this. If successful, you may require professional insurance of some kind. Depending on your location of research, your responsibilities during clinical contact can differ, three common terms are explained in Box 12.1.

If direct clinical contact is not possible, check whether you can participate in departmental meetings, seminars or conferences. In some cities, the opportunity to attend these events are not restricted to the local hospital but also to foundations, pharmaceutical companies and seminars of medical societies.

> **Box 12.1** Typical titles associated with clinical activity overseas
>
> - *Internship*: The student is an active member of a medical team with responsibilities similar to an intern. The student can see patients without the company of a supervisor.
> - *Preceptorship*: The student works with a clinical supervisor, performing and observing all the duties of his supervisor.
> - *Observership*: The students work with a clinical supervisor observing all the supervisor duties but not performing any of them.

## Conclusion

Regardless of your motivation to go abroad, without question it will be a life changing experience. The process of relocating requires lots of time, work, money and perseverance. Professionally, you stand to gain a greatly expanded network and hopefully scientific papers or collaborations. But moving abroad is also an excellent opportunity to explore new cultures: food, music, architecture, traditional excursions… the list is endless. Your colleagues and co-workers are likely to be good sources of information, especially for the more off-piste experiences. On a personal level, through these experiences you will have overcome a range of challenges; adapted to a new culture; discovered skills you might not have known you had; and made new relationships with people from across the world.

## Common pitfalls

1. *'People, especially scientists, are the same everywhere, right?'*
   When moving to a new country it's important you demonstrate respect for your new home, preferably by learning something about it ahead of arrival. Factors like key historic events are helpful to be aware of. On a practical level, know the socially accepted interpersonal space and rules of engagement: some will expect to be hugged, others won't. Other differences might crop up in the work environment such as strict schedules, no social interactions outside working hours or the expectation that you always get involved in institutional activities, like teaching or outreach, even if you are not interested. Do your research and act accordingly.
2. *'My international fellowship is ending soon but I need an extra year of funding to finish my project. Will my supervisor pay during that extra year?'*
   Before and during your project, clarify your funding situation and discuss the different scenarios if there is a gap in funding. This should be done at the earliest opportunity. In a worst-case scenario, international students

without funding can lose their visa. Consult with your supervisors, graduate school and international student office proactively.

3. *'I have concerns with my supervisors, they're acting in a way that does not benefit my PhD training. Who can I turn to?'*

Dual-PhDs abroad are attractive but be aware that in cases of conflict between the student and the receiving institution, it will be more challenging for your programme director at your host institution to mediate and resolve these issues remotely. Refer to Chapter 6 on how to deal with supervisor issues.

## Further reading

1. Mather-L'Huillier, N. Why do your PhD abroad? Available online at the Find A PhD website: https://www.findaphd.com/study-abroad/why-phd-abroad.aspx (Accessed 8 December, 2016).

# Chapter 13 **What I'm really thinking: The post-doc**

*Adel Benlahrech*
Post-doctoral researcher, University of Oxford, UK

## Background

Now that you have embarked on a PhD programme, you are probably aware of the difficulties lying ahead. There is no doubt that completing a PhD program is incredibly demanding, however, if you think that everything will get easier beyond your viva, then think again! The scope of this chapter is not to discourage you from pursuing an academic career but rather to inform you about the realities of the post-doc life and to prepare you for the road ahead.

## It is great to be a post-doc!

If you have decided to follow the academic path, then a post-doc position would be the logical step forwards. It tends to be referred to as research associate, post-doctoral research fellow or simply post-doc and it is typically used as a scientific stepping stone to a permanent academic post. There are many advantages to becoming a post-doc:

- *Research semi-independence*: Generally speaking, the research proposal of a PhD is primarily influenced by the supervisor. Upon taking up a post-doc position you will have greater autonomy and influence on the direction of your research.
- *Reduced teaching and administrative responsibilities*: Unlike post-docs, many academic staff such as lecturers and permanent research staff are required to undertake additional teaching and administrative duties. As a post-doc, this reduced workload gives you the advantage of devoting most of your time to the research you would like to pursue.

*How to Complete a PhD in the Medical and Clinical Sciences*,
First Edition. Edited by Ashton Barnett-Vanes and Rachel Allen.
© 2018 John Wiley & Sons Ltd. Published 2018 by John Wiley & Sons Ltd.

- *Advance your scientific expertise*: As a post-doc you have the opportunity to further your research competency. This can be in the form of acquiring new skills or simply improving on the ones you have gained during your PhD. In addition, many academic institutions now offer personal development programmes which are free or subsidised for post-docs. These include teaching courses, paper and grant writing tutorials, and interview workshops.

## Is it really that great?

Although getting paid to follow your research interests sounds like the ideal job, there are a few disadvantages to being a post-doc which you should be aware of. There are a number of excellent articles published in *Nature* and other journals addressing the issues faced by today's post-docs (see 'Further reading' at the end of this chapter). Below are three of the top difficulties most post-docs meet:

- *Lack of a clear career path*: Many early career researchers think that after obtaining a PhD, a post-doc will automatically turn into a tenured position. Unfortunately, post-docs face an academic bottleneck; there are far too many post-docs and not enough permanent positions. In the UK, it has been estimated that as low as 3.5% of science post-docs become permanent research staff at universities (see Figure 10.1).
- *Lack of job security*: The post-doc period is typically temporary and lasts anywhere between a few months to several years. In most instances, the post-doc position is underpinned by external funding, which makes it highly insecure.
- *Inadequate salaries*: in the UK, the average salaries of post-docs in academia falls below the average of equivalent positions in pharmaceutical industry or even graduate starting salaries for certain professions like banking, law and dentistry. Additionally, due to the nature of research, most post-docs will typically work far more hours than indicated in their job description, which they are not usually financially compensated for.

## A post-doc's advice

You need to decide early on after your PhD what sort of profession you would like to pursue. A post-doc position is not only a stepping stone to becoming a principal investigator. It can also be used to acquire skills for industry jobs and many science-related positions including: medical writing, scientific publishing, project management and public engagement. If your institution provides a career advice or a post-doc development centre, then get in touch with them by all means. For the purpose of this chapter, advice is given to post-docs who are primarily interested in following a typical academic career.

## Choose the position carefully

Many PhD students decide to stay in the same lab as post-docs because they have already invested 3–4 years of their time working on a particular project. Others will stay on because they have a good a relationship with their supervisors and colleagues or simply because it's an easy option. It may also be a daunting task to apply for positions elsewhere while you are still in the process of writing your thesis or preparing for your viva. There is absolutely nothing wrong with staying in the same lab, especially if you want to finish off a paper. However, if you do stay you will most probably be depriving yourself of acquiring new skills and experiences. In addition, at some point in your post-doc career, you will need to start applying for external funding. The funding bodies will find it difficult to determine whether you are capable of conducting your own research in the absence of help from your PhD supervisor. Moving to a different lab will not only demonstrate your independence but will also improve your training and credentials.

## Publications, publications, publications

The most important measure of your scientific achievements is your capacity to publish your research. Your ability to successfully obtain research grants in the future will primarily depend on the volume and quality of your research output. This can take many forms but the most important ones include articles published in scientific journals and abstracts and posters in conferences. Rightly, emphasis is put on primary research articles more so than reviews and abstracts. Your position in the author list is also important; generally speaking, the first author has conducted and probably designed the bulk of the work while the last author has directed, designed, and supervised the work. If you run a PubMed search on most principal investigators in academia, you will most likely find that during their early scientific career their position in the author list tends to be somewhere in the middle. This is followed by a number of first-authored papers during their PhD/post-doc years. Their authorship is ultimately shifted to the last position coinciding with their tenured positions. Thus, during both your PhD and post-doc training, it's imperative to obtain first-authored primary articles if you aim to pursue an academic career. They are arguably less significant if you decide to go into industry or follow non-research based professions. There is evidently no magic number of publications which will guarantee your transition to a permanent academic position, but you need to try and make your CV as competitive as you possibly can. Notably, the quality and impact of your publications are also decisive. You ought to try and publish your work in journals with a high impact factor (IF), which represents the average number of citations to the number of published articles in a given year. It must be noted that it is highly debated whether IF actually reflects how important a journal is within a particular discipline. Alternatively, the impact of your own publications may be reflected by how often they have been cited or whether they have been commended and praised by prominent scientists in your field.

## Grant writing

As a PhD student, you may not appreciate the difficulties your supervisor has to go through to secure funding for your proposed research. Your supervisor would have undoubtedly applied for internal or external grants to cover the full research and administrative costs of your project. You are strongly advised to use your post-doc period as a training ground for grant writing, as you will depend on this skill in your future endeavours, particularly if you go on to become a principal investigator. In fact, your transition to a tenured position is likely achieved through career development fellowships. In the UK, most fellowships are earmarked for post-docs with no more than 6–7 years of experience post their PhD viva. Therefore, it is vital that you do not waste your time and fall into the vicious cycle of 'just one more experiment or just one more paper'.

## Visibility and networking

This does not only apply to your post-doc time, but to all stages of your academic career. A strong professional network is a great source of mentors, collaborators and potential employers. Scientific conferences are a great place to network and become visible. Your visibility can also be increased through online platforms such as Research Gate (www.researchgate.net/), LinkedIn (https://www.linkedin.com), and faculty 1000 (https://f1000.com).

## Teaching and mentoring

More often than not, your life as a PhD student will be influenced by post-docs in your lab. Once you become a post-doc yourself you need to realise that you have a responsibility to look after and guide students in your group. As mentioned earlier, your post-doc time should be used as a training ground for your future academic positions that will undoubtedly require a fair amount of teaching and mentoring skills.

## Conclusion

The life of a post-doc is not all wonderful nor is it all doom and gloom, and it evidently depends on your individual circumstances. Nonetheless, you need to make a decision early on during your scientific career as to what your personal objectives are and plan accordingly. There are many things you can do to make your post-doc life both successful and enjoyable. Make sure you choose your prospective mentor carefully, always publish your research and be as proactive as you can be. You should also surround yourself with like-minded scientists and seek help and advice from all sources available to you. If you have to remember just one piece of advice, this one is probably the one to take on board: Find the right work-life balance that works for you and enjoy your post-doc!

## Further reading

1. Advice to a young scientist by Sir Peter Medawar (Published July 15th 1981). (An excellent guide for early career scientists).
2. Powell, K., The future of the postdoc, Nature. 2015;520(7546):144–147.
3. Rohn, J., Give postdocs a career, not empty promises, Nature. 2011; 471(7336):7.
4. *Science Career Magazine*. Independent Postdocs, Part 1: Gaining Early Autonomy. by Elisabeth Pain, 2009. (Has useful advice for post-docs aiming to gain independence).
5. The Impact Factors of most journals can be found on www.journal-database.com/ and publication citations can be obtained from Web of Knowledge: webofknowledge.com/
6. www.researchgate.net/, https://www.linkedin.com, https://f1000.com are good platforms for enriching your scientific network.

## Chapter 14  What I'm really thinking: The Professor

*Michael Dustin*

Professor of Immunology, University of Oxford, UK

My scientific career spans 44 years out of my 54 on Earth. It started with a chemistry lab passed down from my father to me. He spent his teenage years making explosives and learning some less destructive fundamentals of chemistry, which he passed on informally long before I had a proper chemistry course. This then extended to a photography lab. I feel that early experience with chemistry and using it to make images primed my curiosity and established a useful foundation – quite an advantage when I first entered research labs.

Biomedical science requires a laser like focus and long hours, so it is essential that your area of study resonates deeply with your inner reward system - you need to enjoy thinking about it and feeling in command. The challenge to this pursuit of your interests as a young scientist is identifying the opportunities where your core interests intersect with what is or will be hot in the field, and finding a lab where you have the tools and colleagues to put you in the thick of things. I became fascinated with biological membranes as an undergraduate and then was able to connect with leaders in this area on entering graduate school. Some key advice from a senior colleague led me to the lab of a pioneer in cell-cell communication in the immune system, which provided the desired intersection of my well-developed interests with a hot emerging field.

Taking advantage of opportunities is crucial. When joining this lab, I had the good fortune to inherit a fantastic new reagent that had the potential for innovative findings in many directions. It was not possible to do all of these, but through an excellent training environment with smart colleagues and hard work, I was able to explore a few areas, generate eight lead author papers

*How to Complete a PhD in the Medical and Clinical Sciences,*
First Edition. Edited by Ashton Barnett-Vanes and Rachel Allen.
© 2018 John Wiley & Sons Ltd. Published 2018 by John Wiley & Sons Ltd.

during my PhD, and even more collaborative papers. Reaching these numbers is more difficult in modern biomedical science because of the amount of information that now goes into each paper, but the need to focus on one thing at a time and complete projects before moving on was very important. It also helped to have a well-formed idea of a paper while collecting the data, to do so efficiently, and then to write quickly.

Collaborative science is often the best approach to take on big problems or accelerate research progress. My mentors introduced me to some fantastic collaborators and gave me the freedom to reach out to others. While these connections caused some headaches on occasions, the overwhelming outcome was a fantastic network of colleagues and greater productivity. While these interactions were fantastic, they needed to fit within the framework of a laser focus towards getting things done. Over-commitment is a temptation that must be avoided, at all stages, but most critically in the early years. So, you sometimes need to prioritise and be prepared to say no or 'not now' to new collaborations. Everything takes time!

Looking back over years as a scientist I would say that taking some risks is important – but not everything will work. A challenge in the current competitive environment is achieving a balance between steady productivity needed to sustain the enterprise, and the risk-taking that can lead to bigger payoffs. My thought on this is to have a plan to publish most of the lab work you undertake. As writing scientific papers takes practice, students should be writing more and earlier as a central part of their training. Once in the habit of efficiently experimenting and writing papers in an exciting field, the opportunities and big papers will come with careful thought and hard, enjoyable work.

# Index

---

*How to Complete a PhD in the Medical and Clinical Sciences*,
First Edition. Edited by Ashton Barnett-Vanes and Rachel Allen.
© 2018 John Wiley & Sons Ltd. Published 2018 by John Wiley & Sons Ltd.